BREAKING UP WITH BURNOUT

Identify Your Burnout Pattern, Break the Cycle, and Take Back Your Life

Megan Winkler

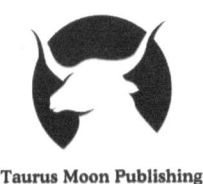

Taurus Moon Publishing

Copyright © 2025 by Megan Winkler All rights reserved.

No portion of this book may be reproduced in any form without written permission from the publisher or author, except as permitted by U.S. copyright law.

This publication is designed to provide accurate and authoritative information in regard to the subject matter covered. It is sold with the understanding that neither the author nor the publisher is engaged in rendering legal, therapeutic, or other professional services. While the publisher and author have used their best efforts in preparing this book, they make no representations or warranties with respect to the accuracy or completeness of the contents of this book and specifically disclaim any implied warranties of merchantability or fitness for a particular purpose. No warranty may be created or extended by sales representatives or written sales materials. The advice and strategies contained herein may not be suitable for your situation. You should consult with a professional when appropriate. Neither the publisher nor the author shall be liable for any damages, including but not limited to special, incidental, consequential, personal, or other damages.

Printed in the United States of America
Digital ISBN 979-8-9987783-0-8
Paperback ISBN 979-8-9987783-1-5
Hardcover ISBN 979-8-9987783-2-2
Published by Taurus Moon Publishing
Little Elm, Texas

Table of Contents

Part II

The Experience of Burnout

Part III

Breaking Up With Burnout

To the rule breakers, the question-askers, the girls who skinned their knees running with the boys on the playground, the girls who wanted to be astronauts and firefighters, and every woman who has refused to accept what we're told we "should" do without first asking why.
Keep challenging the status quo.

The Anti-Introduction: Because Who Has the Time?

(Trust me, you should read this)

Girl, you are worn out. Exhausted by this crazy world we live in—hustlin' for the Benjamins, trying to maintain a social life, nurture your relationships, keep up with your bills, care for your human or fur babies, make it to the gym, stay hydrated, and somehow *also* be a good person. It's too much.

I've been there.

As women, we've been conditioned to believe that enduring stress—both the minor, everyday kind and the huge, life-altering kind—is just part of the deal. We're not taught to thrive in the face of stress, mind you. We're taught to *survive* it. To endure. To sacrifice ourselves for it. Like Pavlov's dogs, we've learned that keeping in line, going with the flow, and acting like "good girls" means we'll be rewarded and avoid negative consequences. And for the most part, this works just fine for the larger machine that is society. *Until it doesn't.*

I learned that the hard way.

My Breaking Point

In 2021, at the height of COVID-19 related chaos, my stress survival skills finally hit their limit. The pandemic was a boon for my online business. I was working harder than ever before. My partner's job—already a remote position—was also busier than ever. With everyone online for pretty much everything, my marketing business and his data security position were in high demand. Needless to say, the pressure to work harder, serve my clients, hold the family together, avoid doom scrolling, and make sure my son kept up with his remote high school curriculum had made me like Mount St. Helens, ready to explode. I just didn't realize it.

Then one random Sunday morning, standing in line at a local brunch spot, it all came boiling up.

At first, it was just small talk with another couple. My partner complimented the wife's hat (*he's a big hat guy!*). Then, out of nowhere, the husband launched into a rant about masks, pandemic restrictions, and all the usual anti-science nonsense. What he didn't know was that one of our closest friends had just been diagnosed with a serious heart condition caused by COVID-19. This friend—once young, thriving, and healthy—would never be the same. They struggled to walk across a room without getting winded.

And this guy just wouldn't shut up. He'd found his soapbox, jumped on it, and wouldn't back down. It was like a Rush Limbaugh nightmare happening right before my eyes. The restaurant manager, whom we've known for years, came over to see what was up and asked the guy to leave. My husband was, rightfully so, standing up for us. The wife was trying to get her husband to chill.

But the longer he ranted, the more I felt the walls closing in. My hands shook. My vision blurred. I wanted to escape. And then—out of nowhere—I started *crying*. Right there. In the middle of a packed restaurant.

This was not me. I don't cry in public. I don't make a scene. I keep things together. Except, in that moment, I was the opposite of together. I was completely unraveling. I couldn't stop my body from trembling. I could barely string words into sentences, babbling nonsense while my vision blurred at the edges. I was having a full-on panic attack, something I'd never experienced before. And I didn't even understand why.

That's the tricky thing about burnout—it sneaks up on you. I *thought* I was just handling life. I *thought* I could push through. But burnout doesn't care what you *think*. It was already at work, slowly eroding my resilience, leaving me fragile and emotionally raw. And this one random brunch confrontation was my breaking point.

I'd pushed myself beyond my capacity to the point that I just sort of broke. The anti-masker wasn't the problem, just an outside stressor that proved to be the last straw. I'd become incapable of coping with the stress in my life.

Burnout Is a Women's Issue

Ask a woman what burnout is, and she might struggle to define it. But ask her if she's felt it? She won't hesitate.

For some women, burnout looks like over-performing at work, diving head-first into a "live to work" mentality. For others, it looks like detaching from society, scrolling TikTok for hours, or numbing out with another glass (or three) of wine. And for some, it looks like barely treading water—just focusing on whatever is immediately in front of them, too overwhelmed to think beyond the next task.

Zero judgment for any of these states, by the way. I've known my share of 15-hour workdays, mindless, wine-fueled social media scrolling, and days when I looked like a deer in the headlights, thinking about nothing but the long to-do list right in front of me.

I've lived all of these burnout states. And I bet you have, too.

The fact that burnout feels inevitable—almost *expected*—for women is exactly why we need to talk about it. The causes and effects of burnout go far beyond the workplace. They seep into our relationships, our emotional well-being, and our sense of self. Burnout doesn't just make us tired—it disconnects us from our own lives.

Burnout keeps us small. It keeps us too tired to fight back, too overburdened to ask for more, and too disconnected from our own power to demand something different. It convinces us that this is just the way life is—that if we can't handle it, we must be weak, lazy, or failing in some way. But what if that's not true?

What if burnout is not a personal failing, but a byproduct of a system designed to keep women depleted?

Breaking Up With Burnout Is a Radical Act

In the process of burning out—and sometimes in an effort to prevent it—we build protective barriers between ourselves and the world. Maybe that looks like putting on extra weight as a subconscious form of armor. Maybe it looks like avoiding friendships with other women to escape the unspoken competition we've been conditioned to feel. Maybe it looks like keeping ourselves so busy that we never have to sit with the real question: *What do I actually want?*

No matter what form it takes, burnout robs us. It steals our energy, our time, and our ability to imagine more for ourselves.

Breaking up with burnout isn't just about feeling better—it's about reclaiming our lives. It's about stepping out of the systems that were designed to keep us small and stepping into a life that prioritizes our needs, our desires, our joy.

And when we do that? We don't just change our own lives. We change the world around us.

By doing this personal work—by de-normalizing burnout—we begin to dismantle the systems that depend on women being overworked and under-supported. One woman setting boundaries ripples outward, showing others that it's possible.

One woman prioritizing rest instead of constant productivity starts a conversation. One woman reclaiming her time makes space for another to do the same.

The result? A more equitable world.

A world where women are paid fairly, valued for more than just their output, and given the actual freedom to choose how they want to live. A world where we have time, space, and energy for the things that bring us joy—not just the things that keep us afloat.

Burnout is not a personal problem. It's a collective one. And breaking free from it is not just self-care—it's resistance.

This book is your roadmap.

How I Got Here (a.k.a. Why This Book Exists)

My own case of burnout was acute. Through therapy, anti-anxiety medications, and intentional recovery, I was able to move out of the cycle. But chronic, year-after-year burnout is a reality for many women. I see it in my friends, my clients, and even in my own family. As long as we perpetuate burnout as normal, we will continue to be hogtied by forces larger than ourselves.

When the smoke cleared, and I finally had the energy to do something about it, I did what I do best: I researched the hell out of burnout.

One of the biggest lessons from my master's degree in military history (yes, really—plot twist!) was learning how to strip away bias when analyzing the past. People assume that history is just a collection of stories, but in reality, it's a discipline rooted in evidence, patterns, and causation. A historian's job is to connect the dots without letting personal bias dictate the narrative.

So, I took that same historian's mindset and applied it to my own burnout. I wanted to know *why* it happened—not just to me, but to women *everywhere*. Because if we understand the reasons behind a problem, we can break the cycle.

As I dove into the research, one glaring truth became impossible to ignore: the science of burnout, like so much of medical and psychological research, was never designed with women in mind.

Burnout studies began in the 1970s, a time when women could still legally be fired for being pregnant. The workplace wasn't built for us, healthcare wasn't designed with our bodies in mind, and the systems we live within continue to squeeze every last drop of energy from women before offering them solutions that amount to *"have you tried self-care?"* The deeper I dug, the clearer it became: burnout isn't just personal—it's systemic.

But I didn't stop at the research. I went inward.

I knew I couldn't intellectualize my way out of burnout (trust me, I tried), so I turned to healing. I read every book I could find on stress, trauma, and the unique pressures placed on women. I dove into neuroscience and meditation studies. I learned more about Internal Family Systems (IFS), a transformative therapy model that I'll introduce you to in this book. I trained as a Reiki Master. I developed a tool called the Energy Management Profile, which helps people align their strengths with their natural energy rhythms to redefine productivity on *their* terms.

And somewhere in the middle of all that, I got my MBA—because, apparently, I don't know how to rest. Later, when we dive into the different types of burnout, you'll see why this didn't push me over the edge. My threshold for mental input is much higher than, say, my capacity for empathic stress.

Through it all, a picture began to form: burnout isn't just about overworking. It is about *over-giving, over-performing, and over-functioning* in systems that demanded more than we were ever meant to give.

So, what do you do when you piece together a giant puzzle and realize the whole damn system is broken? If you're me, you write a book.

Because this information needs to be out in the world. Because I've seen the way burnout drains incredible, brilliant women of their energy, creativity, and joy. Because I refuse to let burnout be the status quo or a badge of honor. We need a new way forward—one that doesn't require us to sacrifice ourselves in the name of productivity, perfection, or keeping the peace.

Burnout Is More Than a Buzzword

When I first started researching burnout, I received a lot of feedback about how popular the term had become. No one has accused me of jumping on a trend, which is nice, and I have to acknowledge that there's a certain amount of trendiness to burnout education and solutions. Why is that?

Over the past few years, we have become hyperaware of our health—both physical and mental. Even before the COVID-19 pandemic, burnout was rampant. But it wasn't always obvious. In fact, it was often glorified. There was this certain pride that came with being a workaholic, in pushing past exhaustion, in "doing it all." Then March 2020 happened. Suddenly, the world locked down, and we became painfully aware of our mental health. When all the sourdough bread was baked, the dog walked for a third time in a day, and the virtual workday done, we had to sit with our internal monologues about what was important. And we were also going through collective trauma at a global scale.

For many of us, the pandemic forced a stark realization: we could exchange simple emails instead of sitting in endless meetings. Without constant workplace distractions, we could accomplish eight hours of work in just five and a half. We saw just how much money we saved—on childcare, gas, work clothes, and daily coffee runs. And perhaps most surprisingly, we rediscovered hobbies, simply because, for the first time in a long time, we had nowhere else to go and nothing else to do.

So yes, talking about burnout became trendy. Largely because we couldn't look away from it anymore. It was right there, in our faces. Burnout is an epidemic—and the good news? It's a treatable one. It doesn't always take therapy either. What it does take is a deep connection to yourself and a dedication to making things better.

What To Expect from This Book

Through my research, the writings and teachings of women doing work in related fields, coaching my clients, and my own healing journey, I started identifying patterns. I saw that burnout wasn't just one thing—it wasn't just exhaustion or just overwhelm. It manifested in different ways, affecting people differently depending on their personalities, environments, and emotional capacities. That's when I developed the framework at the heart of this book:

Burnout isn't one-size-fits-all. There are six different types of burnout, and most of us experience a mix of them.

Recognizing your unique burnout pattern is the first step to breaking free. If you don't know how burnout is showing up in your life, you can't stop it.

Burnout recovery isn't just about rest—it's about restructuring your life. Once you know what's burning you out, you can make strategic changes to prevent it from creeping back in.

This book is about reclaiming your freedom from burnout and reshaping your life in a way that supports you. It's about mitigating stress before it breaks you and not just surviving, but thriving. It's about breaking harmful patterns and healing generational cycles that have kept women locked in a system that does not serve us. And perhaps most importantly, it is about creating space for joy, for creativity, for better decisions in all aspects of life.

We get to explore our own desires, not just the ones society has conditioned us to chase. And in doing so, we begin to dismantle burnout—not just for ourselves, but for future generations.

The good news? We live in a world that is *ready* for change. Productivity is being redefined. Work is being reimagined. We have an opportunity to reclaim our time, energy, and well-being—on *our* terms. This book is your roadmap to doing exactly that.

How We'll Get There

First, in Part 1, we'll uncover the root causes of burnout—from the systemic forces that set us up for exhaustion, to the cultural expectations and personal habits that keep us stuck.

Then, in Part 2, we'll explore the six types of burnout so you can recognize your personal patterns and understand how burnout uniquely manifests in your life.

Finally, in Part 3, we'll dive into practical strategies to break free from burnout, rebuild your energy, and create a life that actually supports you—without falling back into the cycle.

This isn't about perfection. It's about progress.

And if at any point this feels overwhelming? Put the book down. Go for a walk, blast your favorite Beyoncé song, or do 20 jumping jacks—whatever helps you shake off the stress. Seriously, this is a practice worth incorporating into your everyday life. A quick burst of movement is one of the simplest and fastest ways to regulate your nervous system and release stress from your body.

This work is simple, but that doesn't always mean it's easy. That's why I wrote this book—to remind you how powerful you are, and to guide you in reclaiming your time, energy, and well-being. You, my friend, are a badass bitch who gets to decide how you're going to live your life.

Are you ready? Let's do this.

PART I
The Roots of Burnout

1

(Re) Defining Burnout

"**N**ow *everyone can be Van Gogh. It's so easy. Just follow the simple instructions, and in minutes, you're on your way to being an artist,*" recites Connie, a student in the film *Mona Lisa Smile*, as she reads from the side of a Paint-by-Numbers kit. Another student, Giselle Levy, responds, "*Van Gogh by numbers?*" to which their professor, Miss Katherine Watson, remarks, "*Ironic, isn't it? Look at what we've done to the man who refused to conform his ideals to popular taste, who refused to compromise his integrity. We've put him in a tiny box and asked you to copy him.*"

Mona Lisa Smile tells the story of Katherine Watson, played by Julia Roberts. Watson is an art professor who accepts a teaching position at Wellesley College. It's one of my favorite movies about feminism, because it pits Roberts's Watson against the very opinionated and super-conservative Betty Warren, played by Kirsten Dunst, who is simply, deliciously awful. She's a true antagonist who elicits both sympathy and frustration—you feel sorry for her as she's caught in the fishbowl of a conservative upbringing, yet at the same time, you want to see her fail because she writes nasty editorials about women on campus who defy traditional standards. The conflict between the two women perfectly illustrates that while, in the 1950s, feminists pushed to break women free from restrictive societal roles, true feminism allows for all paths—whether career-driven, family-focused, or something in between.

Watson uses the Paint-by-Numbers Van Gogh lesson to illustrate a broader point about the societal pressures faced by the women she's teaching. Throughout the film, we see these young women grapple with the stress and expectations of being women in a rapidly evolving, post-WWII world—sometimes to the breaking point.

Or do we dare call it the *burnout* point?

The first academic definition of burnout dates back to the 1970s, when American psychologist Herbert Freudenberger used the term to describe the experience of people in high-stress "helping" professions, such as doctors and nurses. Freudenberger observed that these professionals often became exhausted and unable to cope with the relentless demands of their jobs, so he sought to understand the phenomenon.[1]

I can't help but notice the correlation between the "helping"

---

1. "Depression: What Is Burnout? - Informedhealth.org - NCBI Bookshelf," InformedHealth.org (Institute for Quality and Efficiency in Health Care (IQWiG), June 18, 2020), https://www.ncbi.nlm.nih.gov/books/NBK279286/.

professions in Freudenberger's work and the conditioned role of women as primary caregivers and even "helpmeets" to their husbands. As a society, we expect so much from women —as mothers, friends, and employees—that something inevitably suffers. Too often, it's the women themselves who bear the cost.

Until now, burnout has been defined by three core symptoms, primarily in relation to the workplace. However, it's clear that the pressures surrounding us—not just as professionals, but as humans, and particularly as women— contribute to burnout in profound ways. And with these varied causes comes a broader range of symptoms that extend beyond the clinical definition of burnout as we know it.

Let's start there, though.

Clinical Symptoms of Burnout

The three most common symptoms of burnout include exhaustion, alienation from activities, and reduced performance.[2] Again, these symptoms are framed in the workplace context, but, as I've stated, burnout takes many forms and can happen in any part of our lives—especially in the 21st century.

---

2. Ibid.

In this model, burnout's three symptoms are:

1. Exhaustion
2. Alienation
3. Reduced performance

I know you're familiar with exhaustion, the first of the three symptoms. We're exhausted when we're drained physically or mentally. Sometimes it feels as if we'll never catch up on sleep! Exhaustion also brings physical issues, from stomach problems to headaches.

The second warning sign of burnout is alienation. When we're burned out, we feel alone. We're convinced we're the only ones who have ever experienced this kind of stress. This often leads to self-isolation. Alienation in work activities can manifest as cynicism about colleagues and working conditions. It can also cause emotional distance and a detachment from the results of our work.[3] If you've ever hit that *"I just don't care"* point, this will resonate.

Finally, there's the reduced performance associated with burnout. Not only do we become apathetic about our work, but we also become less productive and effective because of it. We lose motivation and can't be bothered to put in the effort we once did.

Like the definition of burnout, our ideas of what productivity and work should look like need to shift as well. After all, some of the most burned-out people today are stay-at-home

---

3. Ibid.

moms. There's a ton of unpaid labor—emotional, physical, and mental—that goes into being a stay-at-home parent. Believe me, I've been there. It's time to redefine and broaden our understanding of burnout and its causes.

Stress, Burnout, and Depression

It's important to remember that burnout has a lot in common with both depression and stress. In a way, they're like three terrible muses, overlapping and feeding off each other's energy. As I've stated, the most fundamental symptom of burnout is complete exhaustion. When we're burned out, we've moved beyond everyday stress—no evening off, weekend away, or even vacation can fully restore us.[4] The kind of exhaustion that resists normal stress relief techniques is deeply disturbing. Having been there myself, I know first-hand how it feels—like the world will come to a screeching halt if *you* don't do the things you *have* to do.

But how does that differ from chronic stress?

According to the American Psychological Association, chronic stress is a persistent state of stress that lasts for an extended period. It can feel overwhelming and significantly impact both physical and mental health. Some of the problems that come with chronic stress include muscle pain, high blood pressure, a weakened immune system, insomnia, and

---

4. Bryan E Robinson, "The Surprising Difference between Stress and Burnout," Psychology Today (Sussex Publishers, November 18, 2020), https://www.psychologytoday.com/us/blog/the-right-mindset/202011/the-surprising-difference-between-stress-and-burnout.

anxiety. It can also contribute to major illnesses like obesity, heart disease, and depression.[5]

While long-term stress can lead to burnout, regular day-to-day stress can actually be good for us, serving as motivation to be, act, and do better. Short-term stress helps us push forward and achieve our goals. But there's a tipping point—too much stress stops being helpful and becomes harmful.

It's all really fuzzy, isn't it? The scholarly work on burnout mostly focuses on the workplace, making it difficult to define burnout beyond work performance. Is it chronic stress if it's unrelated to work? Or is it burnout if it stems from a career? You see the problem.

Thankfully, I'm not the only one who thinks ignoring non-work-related burnout is a bad idea. Emerging research is addressing this deficiency by highlighting personality traits and general life factors that may play a role in burnout. For instance, a 2021 study conducted in France, Spain, and Switzerland found that schoolteachers experience burnout due to far more than just on-the-job stress. The study identified several predictors of burnout, including:

- Sex
- Age
- Unreasonable work demands

---

5.   Jennifer F Kelly and Helen L. Coons, "Stress Won't Go Away? Maybe You Are Suffering from Chronic Stress," American Psychological Association (American Psychological Association, October 25, 2019), https://www. apa.org/topics/stress/chronic#:~:text=But%20chronic%20stress%2C%20which%20is,and%20a%20weakened%20immune%20system.

- Weekly working hours
- Autonomy in one's job
- Support in the workplace
- Sentiments of accomplishment
- Leisure activities outside of work
- Support in one's personal life
- Non-work-work conflict[6]

You don't need a degree in psychology to see that these factors span the work and non-work aspects of our lives. In fact, the researchers stated that de-emphasizing individual and non-work factors is harmful—a conclusion I wholeheartedly agree with.[7]

Yet, the burden of expanding burnout research falls on individual scholars. Unfortunately, companies care most about workplace productivity, so they fund studies that focus on work-related burnout. As a result, the research remains limited, reinforcing a narrow view of burnout. Until we push for research that explores burnout across all aspects of life—and considers a diverse range of people—we'll lack the information needed to create a more equitable society. We'll also be stuck in a pattern of burnout like the one we're in now.

For now, we've got to pave our own way through this forest. To start, let's remember that:

---

6. Renzo Bianchi, Guadalupe Manzano-García, and Jean-Pierre Rolland, "Is Burnout Primarily Linked to Work-Situated Factors? A Relative Weight Analytic Study," *Frontiers in Psychology* 11 (January 13, 2021), https://doi.org/10.3389/fpsyg.2020.623912.
7. Ibid.

The difference between burnout and even chronic stress isn't so much about where we're experiencing it but about whether or not recovery is possible. When chronic stress becomes unmanageable or unrecoverable, it turns into burnout.

It's also important to remember that there's nothing wrong with you if you're experiencing burnout. It has become so common. A big reason for that is the world isn't made for women (a topic we'll be diving deep into in the next few chapters)—and we're changing that! In the meantime, there's a lot of adjusting and shifting, which, of course, is going to stress us all out, so we've got to remember we're in a marathon, not a sprint.

Burnout Levels Are Rising Among Women

Studies show that 53% of women report higher stress levels than in previous years. In one such study, nearly half of the women surveyed reported feeling burned out.[8] It makes sense to me. Women hold the world up on their shoulders. We're caregivers—even if we don't have children. We're the ones who pick up the household chores more often. The ones who make the doctor appointments, get the dog to the

8. Michele Parmelee, "Deloitte Brandvoice: Women Continuing to Face Alarmingly High Levels of Burnout, Stress in the 'New Normal' of Work," Forbes (Forbes Magazine, April 27, 2022), https://www.forbes.com/sites/deloitte/2022/04/26/women-continuing-to-face-alarmingly-high-levels-of-burnout-stress-in-the-new-normal-of-work/?sh=426ccad7432e.

vet, make sure there's food in the fridge...you know this. You're there.

And here's the thing: we didn't get here by accident. Society has conditioned us to believe this is what will bring us happiness. The idea of "having it all" has been propagated by marketing firms for decades.

In the climactic scene of *Mona Lisa Smile*, Katherine confronts her class after Betty—who's sitting in the room—writes a damning editorial about Katherine's challenge to *"the roles you were born to fill"* as women. Katherine, full of justified anger, projects a series of advertisements on the screen at the front of the class.

"What will future scholars see when they study us? A portrait of women today?" Katherine asks. She continues to deliver her speech to the class, culminating in an image of an ad with the headline:

"A girdle to set you free."

"What does that mean?!" she yells at the class and to the projection screen.

What *does* it mean? I think what she's asking is: what does *any* of this mean?

2

The Patriarchal Roots of Burnout

I'm using buzzwords in this book to disconnect the "buzz" from the word's actual meaning. One of those words is *patriarchy*. At its core, patriarchy simply refers to a society or government set up in which the male members of society are viewed as the default human. It's a system that is set up for the benefit of men, and our family lineage is defined through male descendants. It's one reason that, until recently, women typically took their husband's last name.

However, during Katherine Watson's time, when women like her were asking, *"What does it all mean?"* the lines between the genders were far more rigid. And while we have made progress as a society, we still hold on to much of that patriarchal conditioning. Men continue to dominate corporate leadership. The wage gap persists. We still haven't had a woman president, and the 2024 race isn't looking good for us ladies.

As we attempt to understand how we got here—because having a firm grasp on what led us here will help us heal—let's look at the historical roots of patriarchy, gender roles, institutional power, cultural norms and media, and intersectionality. We're dealing with a whole system that's unsupportive of our needs and desires as women, and it's within this system that burnout thrives.

The Herstory of the Patriarchy

For thousands of years, we've been told that we are less than men, need to have a man tell us what to do, and need to adopt male attributes in order to succeed. We've seen it in movies, books, and advertisements that claim a razor (or a girdle!!) will free us from...something. How often have you seen a woman who burns out trying to fit into the metaphorical man's suit—adopting his ways of doing business or leading a team? How often do our daughters struggle with the idea that they are less valued than boys?

Over time, these attitudes about male-dominance permeated our halls of government. What began as a way to keep property and power within families became the default method of rule. Long before marriages were based on love, and centuries before DNA tests, the only way to ensure a legitimate line of succession was by restricting the behavior of noble women. This is one reason Queen Elizabeth I never married—staying single allowed her to maintain full sovereignty over herself.

Motherhood, after all, is indisputable—a baby pops out of her body and, the more noble the woman, the more public the birthing process was. There are actual accounts of queens and princesses being surrounded by male advisors and lawmakers to ensure the baby (*ahem*) presented was the same baby that was named as the heir.

Fatherhood, on the other hand, was far less provable. So, men could go about their merry way, sowing their seeds as they pleased, while women were expected to remain chaste and controlled to ensure that when the time came to produce an heir, there was no question that the child was, in fact, the rightful offspring of her husband.

Fast-forward to the 20th century, and we see that our advancements toward equality are still relatively new. Younger generations may take some of these advancements for granted, but many of them were won just a generation or two ago. For instance, the Equal Pay Act was passed in 1963. President Nixon signed the Education Amendments of 1972, including Title IX, which prohibits academic discrimination based on sex. In 1981, Sandra Day O'Connor became the first woman to serve on the Supreme Court.[1]

That was the year before I was born. This is recent history.

It wasn't until 1974 that women could finally apply for and receive credit in their own names, thanks to the Fair Credit Reporting Act.[2] And as late as 1988, the Women's Business

1. "Women's Rights Timeline," National Archives and Records Administration (National Archives and Records Administration, June 17, 2022), https://www.archives.gov/women/timeline#event-/timeline/item/sandra-day-oconnor-becomes-first-woman-to-serve-on-the-supreme-court.
2. Erica Sandberg, "The History of Women and Credit Cards," Bankrate, March 8, 2022, https://www.bankrate.com/finance/credit-cards/history-of-

Ownership Act finally allowed women to take out business loans without a male relative's signature.[3] Even now, we're still fighting to protect the progress we've made—battling legal rollbacks on reproductive rights, gender equality, and marriage access.

Sushi Rolls, Not Gender Roles

The bigger challenge in our modern world is that power remains concentrated in the hands of a select few. Even in the representational democracy of the United States, the voices of everyday people are often overlooked in favor of political and corporate interests. What most average Americans truly want and need is frequently ignored by those in power—who, more often than not, are men.

I live in Texas, so I've had to live with the actions of some fiercely undesirable men making decisions for me. Texas is one of the many gerrymandered states in the U.S., which means that in some regions, the dissenting vote carries less weight than it should. This is why we've ended up with the likes of Ted Cruz, the senator we all love to hate.

But it's not just men keeping this system in place. Within government, we have far too many women willing to vote

---

women-and-credit-cards/#:~:text=1974%3A%20The%20Fair%20Credit%20Opportunity%20Act,-It%20-
took%2016&text=In%201974%2C%20the%20Fair%20Credit,%2C%20na-tional%20origin%E2%80%94and%20gender.
3. Valerie Rein, *Patriarchy Stress Disorder: The Invisible Inner Barrier to Women's Happiness and Fulfillment* (Austin, TX: Lioncrest Publishing, 2019), 42.

against their own well-being. Republican lawmaking women will vote against the rights of their own gender in the name of securing political power. Of course, because many of them come from a place of privilege, they'll never suffer the consequences of their own policies. If they or their daughters need reproductive healthcare, for example, they'll be able to afford such services and avoid penalties from their state.

Okay, but how did this happen? Gender roles, baby!

Patriarchal societies enforce general roles. Men are expected to be the providers, leaders, and bosses, while women are expected to take on more domestic and caregiving roles—even in professional spaces. Women are then blocked from making decisions that could lead to generational wealth, education, and political participation. And, ironically, it's often the same domestic and submissive image that some women in politics use to secure votes.

It's easy to become complicit in our own gender-conforming roles because we're rewarded for it. How often do we see women being praised for being soft and feminine—while women who assert themselves are labeled as aggressive, difficult, or unlikable? The media has always reinforced these expectations. Just look at Kate Middleton and Meghan Markle.

Kate is praised for her grace, beauty, and respect for Great Britain, royal protocol, and tradition. Meghan, on the other hand, a "loud" American who stands up for herself, is treated like a pariah by the British media. Part of that is due to racism, which shouldn't go unacknowledged, but part of it is also the way we police women's behavior.

In their 2022 documentary, Harry & Meghan, the Duke and Duchess of Sussex, recounted how Meghan experienced depression so severe that she considered self-harm. Her husband decided it was time to save her from the same fate his mother, the beloved Princess Diana, suffered at the hands of the media and public.[4]

This isn't just a problem for the famous and powerful—it's something women everywhere experience. The pressure to be likable, to conform to outdated gender roles, and to put everyone else's comfort above their own is relentless. And when women push back? They're punished for it. Whether you're a duchess or an office worker, the message is the same: fall in line, or face the consequences.

The media, pop culture, institutions, and cultural norms that surround us reinforce these gender roles in ways we don't always notice—but we feel their impact every day.

Cultural Norms and the Media

In the press junkets for *Barbie*, Margot Robbie talked about how hard it was to film the rollerblading scene because she felt so exposed while doing it. In the film, Barbie and Ken leave Barbieland and arrive in the real world, rolling down Venice Beach in matching neon outfits. It's the first time that Barbie experiences objectification. She realizes that the president isn't a woman and the Supreme Court isn't all seated with female justices (*if only!*).

---

4. "Harry & Meghan," Netflix, 2022.

In some behind-the-scenes paparazzi shots, you can see Robbie and Ryan Gosling riding on a golf cart to the filming location. He's dressed in full costume, while she's covered up with a long robe, only revealing her costume to film scenes. You can see that she feels vulnerable. And perhaps unironically, the scene reinforces that vulnerability for all of us. It's the first time Barbie feels self-conscious, and it rocks the foundation upon which she's always thought about women and the world.

This is a prime example of the many undercurrents in society that burn women out. When we don't have the freedom to be ourselves—because we're worried about being catcalled, groped, or fired—our stress levels rise, as does our likelihood of burnout.

Institutional Marginalization

Trauma follows family lines for generations. Scientifically, this is called epigenetics. We can train rats in a laboratory to fear electric shocks when they smell cherry blossoms, and their offspring will fear the same smell without ever having experienced a shock firsthand. So, too, do we carry the trauma of the generations that came before us.[5] While the trauma didn't start with us, and it isn't "ours" in the sense that it didn't happen to us firsthand, it nevertheless impacts us today.

For our mothers, grandmothers, and great-grandmothers, it was safer to comply. Blending in, following the rules, and not

5. Ibid., 42-44.

talking back was safer. Generations of women learned that challenging the system was dangerous—and that belief has been passed down, even if the world has changed. This is one of the big reasons burnout affects women so deeply—its roots stretch back through generations.

The same goes for the idea that if we just work harder, put in more hours, and pay our dues, we'll be successful. But this belief doesn't account for the invisible barriers in place—not to mention the outdated mores dictating what a woman *should* be and do, and what she *shouldn't*.

These expectations are reinforced by institutions of power. Governmental bodies, school districts, churches—many of them still uphold systems designed to marginalize anyone who doesn't fit the mold of white, male, and Christian.

And as the lines between Christianity and politics blur more and more each year, the first people to suffer are women and the LGBTQIA+ community. But suffering doesn't always come in the form of a single, catastrophic event—it's often a slow erosion. A constant, exhausting negotiation of our place in the world. Whether it's fighting for bodily autonomy, economic opportunity, or even just the ability to exist without scrutiny, these systems don't just hold us back—they wear us down.

Intersectional Considerations

Oppression doesn't affect all women in the same way. Race, class, and identity shape how discrimination is felt and who bears the heaviest burden. For some, systemic barriers are frustrating. For others, they are suffocating.

Look, women's empowerment has never been perfect. Not only does it often exclude non-white women, but it also gets convoluted by the patriarchal systems that fear the challenge. White suffragists didn't include Black women in their mission. Today, Trans Exclusionary Radical Feminists (or TERFs) exclude trans women and believe trans women are hurting the women's rights movement.

And of course, feminism itself has been weaponized. Words like *feminazi* have been around for as long as I can remember. And I can't believe I still hear things like, "Oh no, I don't hate men, so I'm not a feminist." Feminism, like *burnout* or *patriarchy*, has become a buzzword and, therefore, lost a lot of its meaning.

Women of Color, members of the LGBTQ+ community, and those from challenging socioeconomic backgrounds face compounded disadvantages from institutions, men, and even women. For a while, when the *bear vs. man in the woods* debate was happening on social media, a variation of the question popped up from Black women. Would they rather be in a meeting with a white man or a white woman? Most said they'd chose a white man because at least with the man, he'd be super aware of the fact that he was in the room with a Black woman.

That stopped me in my tracks. We white women have an uncanny ability to be sneakily racist toward Black women. It's often unintentional, but that doesn't make it any less damaging.

If we're going to address the epidemic of burnout, we also have to acknowledge the ways we contribute to it. That means actively reassessing how we treat Women of Color, LGBTQ+ individuals, and other marginalized identities—both in and out of the workplace—and being willing to do the work to course correct.

Discussing the "Patriarchy" Doesn't Mean Hating Men

"To be honest, when I found out the patriarchy wasn't about horses, I lost interest." — Ken, as played by Ryan Gosling in *Barbie*.

Here's the deal: We're all stuck in the patriarchal system. It's a framework that places men at the center—as both governing individuals and the primary beneficiaries of society's structures. And ironically, it's backfired on them, too.

Despite a world built by and for them, men are told that they shouldn't be emotional, they should be tough, and they should be inhumanly stoic. Of course, the message is really that they shouldn't cry. Emotions like anger and frustration are acceptable for men, while a boy or man who tears up when moved is a "sissy" or a "pussy."

As Amanda Montel writes in her book, *Wordslut*, "If you want to insult a woman, call her a prostitute. If you want to insult a man, call him a woman."[6] While her book is a deep dive into the gender divide in the English language (and

---

6. Amanda Montell, *Wordslut: A Feminist Guide to Taking Back the English Language* (Harper Wave, 2020), 21.

worth a read—it's both entertaining and educational), it doesn't take a linguist to notice how gendered our language is. And it's not just the language—it's the entire landscape of our society.

It's easy to roll our eyes at guys with their "man colds" and "babysitting" their own children. But it's often other women who are reinforcing these stereotypes. We are just as at fault for promoting and maintaining the patriarchy as men are, and it's because we've been taught to! Just Google "old advertisements" and look at the messaging our mothers and grandmothers were immersed in. Look at what our fathers and grandfathers were conditioned to believe about themselves and about women. And more recently, you have the whole "trad wife" TikTok trend, which is really hurting our attempts at gender equality.

At its core, patriarchy is a rigid framework—one that dictates what men should be and what women should be, while leaving very little room for the nonbinary folks, by the way. It is a framework that continually discounts women's needs *and women's strengths*. It is a framework that focuses on business stats that can be charted in Salesforce and QuickBooks. It is a framework that makes it funny for trad wife content to go viral and normalizes incel behavior.

And it's this very framework that drives women's burnout.

It's easy to feel consumed by rage over it all, but rage alone won't change the system. So, take a deep breath before turning the page.

3

The System Works Exactly as Intended

One night, deep in what they call the Dark Night of the Soul, I had it out with God.

"Why?!" I screamed in my head with that voice that doesn't require any breath—just passion—to speak. *"Why was I born a woman? I have the heart of a man, so why?"*

I was torn up inside, trying to fit into the little box my religion, my upbringing, and my culture had created for me. But no answer came. And the truth is, I wasn't born with the heart of a man.

I was born with a *heart*. Period. End of sentence.

And it is a heart that is so different from the one I was told I should have. I was told I should be happy to be by my husband's side—to guide him as the righteous one in the relationship, to follow him around the world, and to set my desires and professional goals aside. My duty was to bear and raise children. I was supposed to go to church every Sunday (for three damn hours, mind you) and accept volunteer assignments handed down through the all-male priesthood. Sure, I could help "lead" children and women, but never without male oversight.

Damn, that box was cramped. And every day, it got smaller.

No wonder I cried and screamed at God, demanding to know why He had created me like this—with so much drive, ambition, courage, and stubbornness—yet so little power accepted by the world around me. The world I was in was far narrower than the world outside it.

This feeling—the frustration, the exhaustion, the constant battle to balance expectations—this is what leads to burnout. Burnout isn't just about working too many hours at a job. It's a natural consequence of a system that asks women to do everything, be everything, and expect nothing in return.

I once heard a woman speak on current events and social injustice. She said something along the lines of, *"The system isn't broken. It's working just like they intended."*

And she was right. We are living in a system that was never designed to support us. My religious microcosm was just one part of it.

A Brief History of Time

So much of our world is dependent on the 24-hour clock and the 40-hour work week. And this just doesn't serve most of us, especially us women. Studies have shown that while men essentially have a 24-hour circadian rhythm, women's internal clocks are a few minutes shorter. That's why we tend to go to bed earlier and get up earlier than men.[1] Or maybe that's just conditioning—years of rising before dawn to tend to fussy babies, get a jumpstart on household responsibilities, or squeeze in a workout before the workday begins. Just musing here.

The way we experience time—and how it governs our lives—hasn't always looked like this. In fact, in the 1980s, historian Roger Ekirch found public records noting that in the Medieval era, people had a "first sleep" and a "second sleep." He was researching what nighttime was like before the Industrial Revolution and, having never seen the terms first and second sleep before, Ekirch dove into the concept. He found it mentioned in Italian, Latin, and even in documents from the Middle East, South Asia, Africa, and Latin America. It seems that way back in the 1600s, people all over the world would go to bed around nightfall and then wake up around midnight. During that time, they'd relax by the fire, pray, write, catch up on chores, or have sex. Then they'd go back to sleep until the morning.[2]

It will come as no surprise that this time between sleeps was essentially another workday for women. Many of the domestic chores that didn't get finished during the day were

1. Eric Suni, "How Is Sleep Different for Men and Women?," Sleep Foundation, April 22, 2022, https://www.sleepfoundation.org/how-sleep-works/how-is-sleep-different-for-men-and-women#:~:text=Studies%20have%20found%20differences%20in,bed%20and%20wake%20up%20earlier.
2. Derek Thompson, "Can Medieval Sleeping Habits Fix America's Insomnia?," The Atlantic (Atlantic Media Company, May 10, 2022), https://www.theatlantic.com/ideas/archive/2022/01/medieval-sleeping-habits-insomnia-segmented-biphasic/621372/.

completed then. Because while men's work has traditionally had a clear "on" and "off" switch, women's work never ends.

When the Industrial Revolution arrived in the 1700s, it didn't just reshape labor—it reshaped time itself. Factory schedules, artificial lighting, and, of course, caffeine helped push workers toward a more rigid and regulated understanding of time. The expectation became clear: show up, work efficiently, and produce more. Rest became secondary to productivity.[3]

And here we are, centuries later, still fighting for rest. Worse, we've been conditioned to glorify exhaustion.

Recently, I was sitting at the bar in my favorite disco club—yes, really. It's '70s themed and so cute. I got to talking to the woman seated next to me who bragged about owning her own business. We'll call her "Judy."

Judy manufactures a special type of light bulb popular with football coaches for nighttime practices. (*So Texas, right?*) She explained that because a lot of her suppliers are overseas, she often works through the night. To hear her tell it, she goes days without sleep. She doesn't eat—because she gets so busy—and she's super proud of how far she's come. Honestly, after hearing her brag about all the time, effort, sweat, and tears she puts into her business, I was surprised she was sitting at a bar on a Friday night.

Judy is the embodiment of hustle culture. And in her mind, this level of self-sacrifice isn't just necessary—it's a badge of

---

3. Ibid.

honor. As if sacrificing her health and well-being is proof of her dedication, her worthiness.

But why? Where did we get the idea that working ourselves into the ground is something to be proud of? Part of the answer lies in how we've structured work itself.

If you're a fan of *Downton Abbey*, you'll likely remember a scene in the first season where Matthew and his mother are at dinner with the family. Matthew mentions the weekend and Old Lady Grantham looks confused. "What is a weekend?" she asks, in Maggie Smith's classic, faintly condescending way.

The 40-hour work week has been demonized, often accompanied by calls to *"eat the rich"* who are exploiting us. But, as Old Lady Grantham so artfully illustrates—albeit as a fictional character—the weekend is a relatively modern, and fairly progressive, invention. Henry Ford is credited with introducing the 40-hour work week as a way to take care of his factory workers. Now, don't get me wrong—he wasn't exactly a great guy. But we should remember that there was a time when labor unions weren't even an idea yet and working *only* 40 hours in a week was revolutionary.

Unfortunately, even with modern labor laws, we've simply replaced one form of overwork with another. We're no longer working grueling factory shifts seven days a week, but we've replaced that with hustle culture, the expectation of being constantly available, and the pressure to be everything to everyone. The fight for fair wages, work-life balance, and equality isn't over—it's just changed shape. While there are far more diverse patterns in non-Western cultures,[4] it's important to note that it's the values that are the boogeymen in this particular story.

When cultures value productivity, profit, and efficiency, we see historical patterns of more universal time consciousness. Now, none of these values are evil on their own. It's when we value them over self-care, mental and physical health, and individual human beings that there's a problem.

And this model never accounted for unpaid labor.

For centuries, the official workday has been structured around men's labor, while women's responsibilities—childcare, domestic work, caregiving—have been expected to exist outside of it. Even in households where women work full-time jobs, they still take on the majority of unpaid labor. And yet, we don't question it. We don't ask why the work that keeps society functioning is the least valued.

Because the system isn't broken. It was never designed to work for us in the first place.

The Workplace Is Rigged—And Exhausting

Women aren't just working in the workplace—we're fighting an uphill battle in nearly every professional space. We're expected to perform at the highest level, navigate double standards, and somehow still "play nice." And while workplace burnout is universal, the way women experience it is fundamentally different.

---

4. Ibid.

I recently heard a coach friend of mine say, "Men don't worry about burnout," and she's right. They experience it, sure. But they don't anticipate it, especially not white men. The Western world was created by and for them, so they just don't have the challenges that the rest of us do. They don't experience the same emotional labor that women do. They don't have to worry about getting shot during a traffic stop like Black men do. And—let's be honest—they often have a wife at home picking up the slack (we'll come back to this in a minute).

We don't just deal with demanding workloads—we also carry the weight of proving ourselves, managing perceptions, and battling gendered assumptions about our competence. If a man is assertive, he's a leader. If a woman is assertive, she's difficult. If a man is ambitious, he's driven. If a woman is ambitious, she's aggressive.

This constant awareness of how we're perceived is exhausting. It forces women into a state of chronic vigilance—making sure we're not too outspoken, too emotional, too bossy, too soft. We walk a tightrope, and one misstep can lead to losing credibility, respect, or even opportunities for advancement.

It would be nice if we could just band together, lift each other up, and burn the whole system down, right? But in reality, many women in leadership don't challenge the system—they reinforce it.

When Survival Means Playing by Their Rules

The movie *Mean Girls* was largely inspired by Rosalind Wiseman's 2002 book, *Queen Bees and Wannabees*—a self-help guide for parents of teen girls navigating high school cliques and aggressive social behavior. It was so relatable that Tina Fey turned it into a movie.

And let's be real: No matter how old we are, we never quite escape the Regina Georges of the world. It happens among friend groups and within companies.

Most workplaces assume that when women reach leadership positions, they'll bring a "feminine" perspective—mentoring younger women and serving as role models, much like senior men mentor junior male colleagues. Unfortunately, the research shows us that the opposite is true. If you've ever worked for a "queen bee" type, you know what it's like.

Rather than mentoring junior women, women in leadership often distance themselves from their gender. Not because they hate women—but because they had to assimilate to male-dominated work cultures to get where they are. They had to play by the rules, so they expect other women to do the same.[5] Which looks like defining success based on how much money we make, how many deals we seal, how much effort we put into a project, and how far we're willing to go to achieve our goals at work.

---

5. Belle Derks, Colette Van Laar, and Naomi Ellemers, "The Queen Bee Phenomenon: Why Women Leaders Distance Themselves from Junior Women," *The Leadership Quarterly* 27, no. 3 (January 15, 2016): pp. 456-469, https://doi.org/10.1016/j.leaqua.2015.12.007.

If you've ever had a female boss who seemed harder on you than her male colleagues, chances are, she was a Queen Bee. Instead of opening doors for the women behind her, she was trying to prove that she deserved her place at the table by enforcing the same toxic standards she had to endure.

It's not just about leadership. Even in lower and mid-level positions, we've internalized this "there's only room for one" mentality. If there's only one woman in the C-suite or on the executive team, suddenly, every woman around her becomes competition instead of community. And this is exactly how the system is designed to work.

Because as long as we're competing with each other, we're not challenging the system that keeps us burned out, under-paid, and undervalued.

The Emotional Labor of Work

When a woman takes a job, she's more likely to experience burnout—not because she can't handle the workload, but because of all the extra responsibilities she's expected to take on that aren't in her job description.

In many workplaces—especially male-led organizations—women are still expected to take on non-promotable, admin-istrative, or social tasks that aren't technically part of the job. There's often an unspoken assumption that women should be the ones coordinating social outings, maintaining the break room, or picking up the birthday cake.

This unpaid labor takes two forms. First, there's the literal labor—like making the coffee, restocking office supplies, or keeping the office kitchen clean. The number of times I've seen senior male executives walk right past a full dishwasher and an overflowing trash can while a junior female employee instinctively starts tidying up? Infuriating.

Then there's the emotional labor—the invisible, unpaid, and unacknowledged work of managing relationships, emotions, and workplace harmony. There's an unspoken expectation that women will be the ones to keep the office culture running smoothly. We're expected to organize the potlucks, plan the team-building events, make sure birthdays are acknowledged, and—of course—take the meeting notes (because, apparently, our fingers are just naturally better suited for typing).

Beyond logistics, women are also expected to carry the emotional weight of the workplace. We're the ones who are supposed to soften difficult conversations, de-escalate tensions, and ensure that team morale stays intact. If there's workplace conflict, it often falls on women to be the mediators, the soothers, the fixers. And if we don't? We risk being seen as cold, unapproachable, or not a "team player."

It's not that men can't do these things—it's that the default expectation is that women will. And when you pile all this unacknowledged emotional labor on top of an already demanding job, it's no surprise that workplace burnout hits us harder.

One of the biggest pieces of advice I give to women starting their careers is: Don't let people take advantage of you or put extra work on you because you're a woman. Make the coffee in the morning if you love getting that piping hot first cup yourself. Organize the event if the event was your idea and it excites you. But don't let them tell you it's your responsibility if it's not in your job description. The time and energy women spend on unpaid office labor could (and, dare I say, should) instead be spent building their careers, negotiating raises, or leading projects that actually get them promoted.

Workplace Myths That Keep Us Stuck

And then, there's the myth that men and women can't just be colleagues.

We've all seen it: A man and a woman work closely together, and suddenly, people assume there must be something going on. As if they have to *ahem* be doing each other to want anything to do with one another in the workplace.

Here's an example: My beloved partner is a man who often works with women. For a couple of years, he had a female sales partner who was about 20 years younger, and there were all these rumors about them at work. At first, it was assumed that they *had* to be sleeping together. They weren't. Then, when people realized it wasn't that kind of relationship, they assumed that she was his daughter (Because, you know, it couldn't just be a normal work partnership.)

What's notable about this is that if they had been the same gender—two men or two women—no one would have questioned their relationship. No one would have speculated about hidden motives or deeper personal ties just because they work well together. But when it's a man and a woman? People feel the need to assign some deeper meaning to it because they can't fathom a professional relationship without hidden motives. And it's wildly unfair to both individuals. It reeks of that whole "sleeping her way to the top" mentality that popped up when women entered the workplace in force. Because let's be honest, there are still way too many myths about how women get ahead at work.

This kind of speculation is exhausting! The constant undercurrent of suspicion surrounding male-female work relationships only adds to the stress of trying to succeed in male-dominated spaces. It's another layer of social burnout that keeps women in a heightened state of anxiety.

Not that men are *completely* immune to workplace rumors—but let's be real, the stakes are often much higher for women.

Marriage, Motherhood, and the Second Shift

Did you know married men are happier and live longer than unmarried men?[6] It's true. And the romantics out there will say that's because love makes them healthier and happier. Honey, you and I both know it's the fact that they have a wife to take care of them emotionally and physically. I have the most independent and helpful partner—he never suffers from a man cold, he does the dishes, he cooks about half the time, he runs errands, and has more energy than three of me would—and I still have to encourage him to see a doctor

---

6. https://www.health.harvard.edu/mens-health/marriage-and-mens-health#:~:text=Married%20men%20and%20mortality,ended%20in%20divorce%20or%20widowhood.

when he's got a persistent cold. Even in the best cases, we women help our men live happier, longer lives.

What about the women?

Here's something that will make you laugh. In the 1980s, multiple studies suggested that men who were married to educated, intelligent women were more likely to die from heart disease than men who married less educated women. I have no doubt that the studies were flawed and wildly biased. After all, we were still close to the days when women couldn't even apply for a credit card on their own. Society still believed that a woman's "place" was at home. So, of course, the studies claimed men were better off with a less intelligent wife. Ugh.

By the 2000s, research finally caught up. Turns out, the opposite is true. The more educated a wife is, the healthier her husband is: his risk of coronary artery disease, high cholesterol, obesity, and other risk factors go down.[7]

I ask again, what about married women?

It turns out that we have to be *satisfied* with our married lives if we want to see health benefits.[8] Interesting, right? When we're in a satisfying, long-term relationship or marriage, then we experience the same health benefits as men in the same

---

7. Ibid.
8. "Marriage Appears to Be Beneficial to Women's Health, but Only When Marital Satisfaction Is High, New Research Shows," American Psychological Association (American Psychological Association, 2003), https://www.apa.org/news/press/releases/2003/09/marital-benefit.

situation. But for men, the simple act of being married carries health benefits.

Thankfully, we have far more rights and freedom than our mothers and grandmothers did. In most cases, we don't have to stay stuck in a situation that doesn't fulfill us or with a partner who doesn't support us. We're gaining equality, but we're still not there yet.

The Second Shift

Women shoulder the burden of unpaid labor in the U.S.—not because of personal choice, but because the system is structured to depend on it. In fact, we're still doing nearly twice the amount of unpaid labor as men. When the pandemic hit in 2020, around 3.5 million women either cut back on work hours or left their paying jobs to take care of all the unpaid household responsibilities. And, without exaggeration, it set us back a generation.[9]

One of the biggest contributors to this situation is the extreme lack of accessible childcare. Without affordable childcare, caregiving responsibilities fall disproportionately on women, increasing their unpaid labor load and making it harder for them to participate in paid work. If we had access to high-quality, affordable childcare, 17% more women would be in the workforce. For women without a college

9. Kathleen Davis, "What Would It Look like If We Started Paying for Unpaid Labor?," Fast Company (Fast Company, March 7, 2022), https://www.fastcompany.com/90725985/what-would-it-look-like-if-we-started-paying-for-unpaid-labor#:~:text=Women%20are%20still%20doing%20on,progress%20back%20by%20a%20generation.

degree, experts estimate that number would jump to 31%. And here's a stat that will make your head spin: When women have access to good, affordable childcare, they earn close to $100,000 more over their lifetime. They also have an additional $30,000 in retirement savings.[10] Feel free to join me in a collective, *"What the actual fuck?!"*

But unpaid labor doesn't just disappear when women have jobs. Substantial research shows that women bear the weight of family responsibilities—*regardless of employment status.* For decades, researchers have studied what sociologist Arlie Hochschild famously termed the "second shift"—the unpaid work women do at home after their paying jobs end. This isn't just cooking and cleaning. It's remembering to schedule the dentist appointments, tracking kids' ever-changing extracurriculars, and planning meals for the week—all while managing their own professional and personal lives.

Even in relationships where both partners are willing to help, the burden of managing and delegating still falls disproportionately on women. It's the difference between doing a task and being responsible for making sure it gets done.

For example, a woman might ask her partner to "help" by making dinner—but she's the one who planned the meals, made the grocery list, and bought the ingredients. A husband might say, "Just tell me what to do!"—which means his wife is still the one carrying the mental burden of keeping track of what needs to be done in the first place. And if a mother

---

10. Ibid.

leaves town for a weekend? She often has to prepare meals in advance, arrange childcare, and make sure nothing falls apart while she's gone.

This isn't true equality. It's project management.

Women aren't just doing the work—they're expected to be the default keepers of everything. And that expectation is exhausting.

The assumption that women should naturally take on care-taking, emotional labor, and household management extends beyond parenting roles. Single women still spend more time on household chores than single men. Women in partner-ships without children often handle more cleaning, meal prep, and emotional labor—even when both partners work full-time. Women with aging parents are more likely to take on caregiving responsibilities than their male siblings.

As you can see—and likely intuitively know—the problem stems from the way we assign responsibility and emotional labor based on gender. The world still assumes women will be the ones to remember, anticipate, and handle the things that keep life running smoothly.

And it starts early. As people who were raised to be women, we were taught to be caregivers. We're given dollies as little girls, whereas boys are given trucks. You know, when you have both types of toys available—without any adult influence—that boys will play with dolls too? And girls will play with trucks.

As children, girls are taught to "go help your mother" in the kitchen. During holiday times, the men all congregate around the television to watch football, while the women and girls are in the kitchen prepping the meal. Now, don't get me wrong, this works out well for many families. But I can't help but ask myself *why* it works out well. What if men were in the kitchen—the *kitchen*, mind you, not standing around the grill—while the women were gathered in the living room talking about the latest celebrity gossip or watching real soccer (not men's)?

When you're constantly managing households, children, and social expectations, it's harder to compete professionally, rest properly, or carve out time for yourself. It's why women earn less, save less for retirement, and are more likely to experience burnout.

And yet, the world still asks: *Why aren't women further ahead?*

The next time you hear that question, the answer is simple: because we're already working double shifts.

Your Husband, The Breadwinner

We know that women tend to gravitate toward degrees in the humanities and care work—think nursing, teaching—while men are more likely to pursue degrees in science and engineering. Female-dominated industries tend to be lower-paying, and yet, we continue to choose them because we like them.

I gotta hand it to my sisters out there—we're much more likely to choose career satisfaction over a higher paycheck.

But why are we more likely to do that than men? It may be as simple as cultural permission.

The patriarchy reinforces the idea that men are the bread-winners and providers for their families. So, the all-too-common assumption is that a woman working in her preferred field, like teaching or medicine, wouldn't be the provider for her family anyway—because her husband is.

And if she doesn't have a husband? Well, she *should*.

There's an unspoken expectation that eventually, she will get married—which means she doesn't need to be focused on building wealth, paying off student loans, or advancing her career at the expense of her family life.

Her husband will handle that.

We see this kind of bullshit reflected in heteronormative marriage traditions here in the U.S. The father walks his daughter—wearing white for sexual purity and spiritual naivety—down the aisle to be handed off to the man waiting at the other end. In the "olden days," this was quite literally a financial transaction. The bride came with her dowry—wealth or property that transferred from her father to her husband at marriage.

UGH. I digress.

But this outdated framework still influences the way women's careers and contributions are perceived. It's why men get promoted for "being ambitious" while women get questioned about whether they plan to have kids. It's why we're expected to take lower-paying, "nurturing" roles instead of climbing the corporate ladder. And it's why women bear the brunt of unpaid labor—even when they work just as much as their male partners.

The Motherhood Penalty

One of the most deeply ingrained myths in our culture is that a woman's greatest achievement is birthing and raising children. This isn't just an outdated belief—it actively shapes policies, workplace norms, and economic structures that limit women's autonomy.

"If a woman has a child, why would she want anything else?" That question underpins so much of how society treats women. But this mindset isn't just frustrating—it's dangerous to women's careers and financial independence. One study found that belief in traditional motherhood roles was the single strongest predictor of opposition to women working—even more than gender, education, social status, politics, or religion.[11]

Here's the reality: women are paid less, taken less seriously, and penalized professionally—simply because of their gender. And that's true whether they have children or not.

But for women who do have children, the penalty is even steeper.

The motherhood penalty is a measurable wage decrease that

---

11. Catherine Verniers and Jorge Vala, "Justifying Gender Discrimination in the Workplace: The Mediating Role of Motherhood Myths," *PLOS ONE* 13, no. 1 (September 2018), https://doi.org/10.1371/journal.pone.0190657.

mothers experience in the workforce. In fact, this penalty means that women with children make less than both women without children and—get this!—men with children. Yep, that's right. When a man becomes a father, his income level goes up. When a woman becomes a mother, her income level goes down.

Why? Because the same myths that glorify motherhood are used to justify workplace discrimination against women.

Women are expected to "naturally" prioritize their families over their careers. They're assumed to be less committed, less available, and less ambitious once they have children—whether or not it's actually true. And workplaces quietly reinforce these stereotypes by pushing women onto the "mommy track"—limiting their opportunities for promotions, raises, and leadership roles.[12]

And these biases don't just show up in traditional workplaces. Even as a business owner, I've noticed the same pattern. When I talk pricing with male colleagues, they almost always try to haggle or undervalue my work. Meanwhile, women—who know firsthand what it's like to be underestimated—rarely question my rates.

And it all comes back to the same outdated assumption: a woman's primary role is to be a mother. If she has a career,

---

12. Louise Wattis, Kay Standing, and Mara A. Yerkes, "Mothers and Work–Life Balance: Exploring the Contradictions and Complexities Involved in Work–Family Negotiation," *Community, Work &Amp; Family* 16, no. 1 (2013): pp. 1-19, https://doi.org/10.1080/13668803.2012.722008.

it's secondary. If she earns money, it's supplemental. If she seeks success, she must not be a "good" mother.

Of course, we know this is bullshit.

Women have always worked, always contributed, always driven change. But as long as these myths remain embedded in our culture, the motherhood penalty will persist—limiting women's opportunities, their income, and their long-term financial security.

When the System is Life-Threatening

While this chapter has focused on how traditional gender roles contribute to burnout, it's critical to acknowledge that, for some women, the stakes are even higher. Not all long-term relationships or marriages are safe. Some are emotionally harmful. Some are physically dangerous.

In researching this section of the book, I found some sobering facts about domestic violence. One in four women and one in nine men experience intimate partner violence—which includes physical and sexual violence, as well as stalking. One in ten women has been raped by an intimate partner. Intimate partner violence accounts for 15% of all violent crime in the U.S.[13] And the effects don't just harm individuals—they ripple across families and communities for generations.

---

13. "NCADV: National Coalition Against Domestic Violence," The Nation's Leading Grassroots Voice on Domestic Violence, accessed January 25, 2023, https://ncadv.org/STATISTICS.

For many women, burnout isn't just about exhaustion from juggling work, home, and relationships. It's about survival in a system that often fails to protect them. Financial dependence, societal expectations, and weak legal protections can make leaving an abusive situation incredibly difficult. When we talk about the need for systemic change, this is one of the most urgent reasons why.

If you or someone you know is experiencing domestic violence, please know that support is available. You'll find a list of resources at the back of this book—because no one should have to navigate this alone.

What Do We Do with This Information?

Burnout isn't just a personal problem—it's a structural one. We didn't get here overnight, and we're not going to fix it overnight, either. However, if we want things to change, we have to start somewhere.

We've spent this chapter breaking down the ways the system is designed to work against women—how workplace structures, unpaid labor, gender roles, and outdated expectations keep us exhausted, overburdened, and undervalued. Awareness alone doesn't dismantle a system.

So, where do we go from here?

We challenge the narratives that keep us stuck. We stop accepting burnout as inevitable. We advocate for policies that support work-life balance. We unlearn the conditioning that tells us we have to do it all.

And, most importantly, we start talking about it.

Burnout thrives in silence. We have to start naming our experiences, setting new expectations, and helping the people in our lives—especially the men—see what we've been conditioned to endure. If we keep carrying the mental and emotional labor of change on our own, nothing shifts. The system doesn't change unless we make it impossible to ignore. And that starts with conversations.

In a perfect world, men would come to us and ask the good questions about how they can support us, empower us, and make the world better. We don't live in a perfect world. Instead, we need to have conversations with the good men in our lives—our partners/husbands, brothers, friends, fathers, and sons. We need to help them understand our experiences, because they just don't.

I can't tell you how many times I've had a conversation with a man about something that's just an everyday thing for us. Many men literally don't get it until they hear it from a woman, because the world is built for them. They haven't experienced anything different. Honest, kind conversation with men who value our input is how we convert allies to our cause. This is how we foster a generation of men who understand that walking closely behind a woman on the sidewalk at night is perceived as a threat to her. It doesn't matter that he's just walking home listening to a podcast. To her, he's the unidentifiable threat.

"James" is a friend of mine—one of the most sensitive men I know—and worked in the service industry for many years. He wrote an account of a similar evening on his Facebook page one day. James lived close enough to the bar where he worked at the time that he could just walk home after work. One night, he was walking on the same side of the street as a woman who was in front of him. He wasn't paying much attention at first, but then realized that she kept looking over her shoulder to keep an eye on him.

In response, he then slowed his pace and moved over to the other side of the street, creating distance between the two of them. She was able to continue her pace and stopped looking over her shoulder. It was an experience that moved him enough to write quite a long post about it. He understood intellectually that women worried about shady men following them at night, but he was horrified to find that he was one of them.

The same is true in the boardroom (and the bedroom, for that matter!). If we don't communicate with the men in our lives, they're not going to get it. Just like if they don't communicate about their experiences, we can't understand either. James had heard stories about women being afraid to walk by themselves at night, but until he was the "suspicious guy" in the situation, it didn't really hit. He's become more observant of his behavior at night as a result.

A conversation may not fix a problem, yet I truly believe communication is the most valuable skill we can develop. And it's through these communications that we can come to understand each other better. It's worth a shot, right?

Of course, having these conversations isn't always easy—especially when we've spent our whole lives being told that speaking up makes us difficult, demanding, or even unlikable.

The Burnout Point

If you've seen the timeless classic, *Nine to Five*, starring Lily Tomlin, Jane Fonda, and Dolly Parton, you know the scene:

"Look, I've got a gun out there in my purse. And up to now, I've been forgiving and forgetting because of the way I was brought up. But I'll tell you one thing: If you ever say another word about me or make another indecent proposal, I'm gonna get that gun of mine...and I'm gonna change you from a rooster to a hen with one shot! Don't think I can't do it!"— Doralee Rhodes, as played by Dolly Parton

I've heard it countless times: A woman seemingly has everything that she has ever wanted—the great job, the loving family, the beautiful home, right down to the adorable dog. And then, one day, something snaps.

Maybe it's after a long day of work when they find themselves crying at the kitchen counter for no apparent reason. Maybe it's in the car, gripping the steering wheel in silence before walking into the house, trying to summon the energy to be present for their family. Maybe it's in the middle of the night, staring at the ceiling, wondering how they got here.

Burnout doesn't just appear overnight. It builds. It accumulates over years of pushing through, over-functioning, and ignoring our own needs. At first, we tell ourselves we're just tired, that a weekend of rest will fix it. But then the exhaustion doesn't go away. We drink more coffee. We tell ourselves to suck it up. We keep checking the boxes—work, family, friendships, health, self-improvement—trying to do it all.

Until one day, we just *can't* anymore.

Elizabeth Gilbert wrote about this moment in *Eat, Pray, Love* —the night she found herself sobbing on the bathroom floor at 3 a.m., realizing that the life she had meticulously built wasn't making her happy. That moment wasn't about one bad day or one big disappointment. It was the result of years of chasing a version of success that wasn't actually hers.

And isn't that what so many of us do? We hustle toward the next milestone, thinking it will bring fulfillment. The degree. The job. The promotion. The relationship. The house. The next thing. And for a while, checking those boxes feels good. But when we never stop to question *why* we're chasing them, we end up deeply exhausted, unfulfilled, and wondering why it still isn't enough. Just like Doralee cited her upbringing as the reason she hadn't retaliated against her boss's harassment, we too, are often held back by our own conditioning.

Some women reach this moment in their 30s or 40s—after decades of stretching themselves too thin. Others feel it much earlier, realizing in their 20s that the version of success they were sold doesn't fit. Either way, the breaking point isn't just about exhaustion. It's about disillusionment.

We were told that if we worked hard enough, if we played by the rules, if we *did it all,* we'd be rewarded. But instead, many of us find ourselves burned out, underpaid, undervalued, and still expected to keep going. To top it off, our mothers and grandmothers can't help us and end up sympa-thizing but ultimately trying to placate us with sayings like, "That's just how it is."

This is the time when some women radically shift their lives. We pack the car and move to the other side of the country. We quit the job. We dump the boyfriend. We adopt another cat. We cut our hair. And yet, nothing changes. Because the real changes aren't external.

Others don't have that luxury—so they suffer in silence, numbing themselves just to get through the day.

The truth is, burnout isn't just about working too hard. It's about chasing things that don't actually fulfill us. It's about the pressure to be everything to everyone while sacrificing ourselves in the process.

And this is where so many women find themselves—staring at the life they worked so hard to build, only to realize it's breaking them.

We tell ourselves that if we just push a little harder, just achieve a little more, just keep going, we'll eventually feel fulfilled. But when the promotions, the degrees, the perfect home, the relationship, the dream job—when none of it fills the exhaustion-shaped hole inside us, we start to wonder... What's wrong with me? Why isn't this enough?

And that, right there, is the lie burnout sells us—that we are the problem. That if we feel drained, exhausted, and unful-filled, it must be a personal failing. That we must be too weak, too sensitive, too incapable.

But here's the truth: You are not the problem. The system is.

Which means you don't have to keep playing by its rules. And that's where we go next.

Because once you see burnout for what it is, you have a choice: Keep trying to survive in a system that was never built for you, or start rewriting the rules.

4

You Are Not the Problem—But You Are the Solution

S tan Lee famously wrote the line, "With great power comes great responsibility." Well, with great *knowledge* comes great responsibility. Now that you understand how we got here, you have the power (and dare I say, the responsibility) to change your own relationship with burnout—and maybe even the systems that created it in the first place.

Taking responsibility for your own burnout starts with a radical act: choosing yourself.

Your authentic self is the version of you that doesn't mask around strangers, doesn't suffocate your desires, and doesn't just go along to get along. The most powerful thing you can do to combat burnout—and disrupt the oppressive systems that fuel it—is to choose yourself.

So, what do you actually want out of life?

That might sound like an easy question to ask, but it gets harder to answer when you dig deeper and ask yourself *why* you want those things. For example, you might say you want to get married and have kids. But why?

I sincerely hope it's because you genuinely want them—not because you were conditioned to believe that's what you should want. Many of us spend our lives chasing expectations instead of desires. And if we want something different from what society or our families told us we should?

We're met with shame.

Shame is one of the biggest forces keeping us disconnected from ourselves. It convinces us we're not enough, that we need to work harder, do more, and prove ourselves in order to be worthy.

But here's the truth: Shame is a liar. And if we're going to break up with burnout, we have to learn how to stop believing it.

Shame, Shame, Shame

One of the best examples of the role that shame plays in our lives is from *Encanto*. In the film, Luisa—the strong, dependable sister—loses her power. She sings one of the most poignant Disney songs I've ever heard:

> *"Under the surface*
> *I'm pretty sure I'm worthless if I can't be of service*
> *A flaw or a crack, the straw in the stack*
> *That breaks the camel's back*
> *What breaks the camel's back?*

It's pressure like a drip, drip, drip, that'll never stop..."

Luisa doesn't just fear losing her strength—she fears losing her worth.

And that's exactly how shame traps us. It whispers that who we are isn't enough. That we have to do more, be more, prove more—or risk becoming worthless. Burnout doesn't just happen because we're overworked. Burnout happens because we're overfunctioning to compensate for shame.

Shame is a powerful, powerful ~~drug~~ emotion. It's addictive, self-perpetuating, and relentless. It convinces us that we have to keep pushing, keep proving, keep performing— because if we stop, we'll fail, disappoint, or be exposed as unworthy. I can't remember the first time I felt shame, because it was always a part of my human experience.

But I can identify my most persistent source of shame: my hair. I have super curly hair. It literally does the Shirley Temple ringlet thing on its own around my face. And my baby hairs are so tiny and cute. I love my hair so much these days. *And* I used to be ashamed of it.

I was talking to my healthcare provider about this recently. Lakisha is a Family Nurse Practitioner and a friend. One of the things that I appreciate about our relationship—aside from the fact that every medical appointment with her starts with a big, warm hug—is that we can have honest conversations about being humans who also happen to be of different races. Lakisha is Black and often speaks candidly about her experience as a Black woman in the world. It's wonderful. Recently, we chatted about our hair.

She said, "I bet you hated it when you were younger, right?"

Yep. I sure did.

"That's what Black girls have to deal with—all the curls, all the criticism that it's messy."

While I acknowledged that the white and Black high school experiences are obviously different, we found common ground: the pretty and popular girls adhered to a European beauty standard. Long, straight, silky hair was the expectation. She agreed and then told me about the locs she's thinking of getting. I love her!

When I hit puberty, my cornsilk waves freaked out. The hormonal shift turned them into an unruly mess—half-curls, random straight bits, and frizz for days. I, of course, didn't know how to handle it, so kept treating it like I always had, which meant that I was the mayor of Frizz City most days. After a disastrous 7th-grade haircut, the class bully and his girlfriend branded me 'Poodle Head.' They chanted it in the hallways on our way to lunch. I was so ashamed of my hair that I wanted to simultaneously cry and punch my bullies in the face.

And that's the thing about shame—it convinces us we're not good enough, not pretty enough, not smart enough, not *enough*. So we double down on trying to prove our worth, our value, our enoughness to a world incentivized to keep us hustling.

How Shame Shapes Our Lives

Shame forces us to shrink. It's an insidious beast, convincing us that we're less-than and unworthy of love, acceptance, compliments, or compassion. Shame follows us into adulthood too. Worse, it is built into the fabric of our society. We're conditioned to stay in our lane, to stick to what we know, to go along to get along. Because step one toe over the line and shame will be there, ready to smack you back into position.

Honey, if someone tells you to stay in your lane, first of all—fuck them. When you started your journey, your "lane" was a small path through the woods. Now, it's a freeway. You get to pick the speed, the direction, the playlist. I'd love to see you cruising in a gorgeous convertible, your hair flying freely, with some amazing tunes blaring through the speakers.

The preeminent scholar of shame is Brené Brown. She recalls that when she started researching shame, she received pushback from all sides. Because no one wanted to think about shame, let alone talk about it. In her book, *Atlas of the Heart*, Brown outlines her 1-2-3s of shame:

1. *We all have it*
2. *We're all afraid to talk about it*
3. *The less we talk about it, the more control it has over us.*[1]

---

1. Brown, B. Atlas of the Heart: Mapping meaningful connection and the language of human experience. Random House, New York, 2021, 136.

How many things gain power by not speaking about them? By not naming them?

In *Barbie,* there's a moment when Barbie says to Ken, "I feel kind of ill at ease, like I don't know the word for it, but I'm... conscious, but it's...myself that I'm conscious of." It's the first time Barbie felt self-conscious and it was so foreign to her that she struggled to describe the vulnerable emotion. Meanwhile, the rest of us in the audience nodded knowingly. That feeling? It's shame. It's the discomfort that creeps in when we sense we're not "doing enough" or when we perceive that we've failed at living up to someone else's expectation.

Shame isn't the same as guilt, though many of us were taught otherwise. I'll dig into guilt (and other burnout emotions) later, but here's what you need to know now: shame isn't just a byproduct of burnout. It's one of burnout's biggest causes. And when shame convinces us we're not enough, we push harder, overextend ourselves, and burn out trying to prove otherwise.

And yet, being shameless is somehow a bad thing? As if we should be embarrassed for celebrating ourselves, dressing to the nines, or speaking our minds. So many of my clients feel shame around promoting their work, pricing their services, or owning their success. Maybe you've seen those social media posts that start with, "Okay, a little shameless self-promotion..." Why do we feel the need to apologize for taking up space? For advocating for ourselves? We've been taught that it's unattractive—even sinful—to talk about our own value, so it seeps into every part of our lives, including our careers.

Shame isn't just something society places on us—it's something we carry within ourselves, shaping our choices and our sense of worth. It seeps into our identities, our relationships, and our faith. And sometimes, it takes years to recognize just how much power it holds over us.

Shame is Personal

One of the biggest turning points in my life came with a ton of shame. To give you a little backstory, I went through a deeply religious phase as a young adult while searching for meaning outside myself—a way to explain the Universe through something that felt acceptable and normal. Being the product of Methodists on one side and Southern Baptists on the other, that search for meaning started within the bounds of Christianity. That meant that I didn't stray too far as an adult, but I did venture into Mormonism.

I joined the Church of Jesus Christ of Latter-Day Saints when I was 19. My boyfriend (who later became my husband, and then my ex-husband) had been raised LDS, and when I started talking to him about it, I was intrigued.

Don't get me wrong—I now fully see how cultish the LDS church is, but at the time, it made sense to me. As I have studied more about cultish behavior and cults like Scientology (don't come for me, Tom Cruise!), I realized that the LDS church shares a lot of the same characteristics. At first, the teachings seem logical, and the commitment doesn't feel overwhelming. And before you know it, you're running church programs for no pay, pouring your time and energy into them as a young mother. The church isn't just a place of worship—it becomes the center of activity and belonging, around which you center your entire life.

So when I made the choice to divorce my husband and became a single mother, I unlocked a whole new level of shame I hadn't expected. My husband hadn't died—that would have come with its own kind of pity. And I hadn't always been a single mom—that was a different kind of shame. Instead, I was a woman who *chose* to leave her husband, the sacrament of marriage, and to raise my child in a "broken" home.

But let me tell you, that home wasn't broken because of divorce—it had been broken long before. We fought like cats and dogs, and our marriage was beyond repair. Still, within the church, I was seen as the problem. A divorcee by choice, with an 18-month-old on my hip? The judgment was relentless. I wasn't just leaving a marriage; I was pushed out of the only community I knew—the place that had once been my spiritual anchor.

One day, in the midst of the process of divorce, I went to Mardel, a Christian book and education store. I sneaked over to the Bible section, feeling like such a rebel for buying a King James Bible to read from instead of the giant, heavy quad publication from the Mormon bookstore. I swear, that thing was so massive, I could have thrown it through a closed window and shattered the glass. Anyway, as I was buying that Bible, I just knew I'd run into someone who could somehow tell I was Mormon and I'd get in trouble. Dear reader, I was *ashamed* to be buying a Bible.

And that's how shame works. It doesn't just make us feel bad about our choices—it reinforces the conditioning that tells us to stay in line, to follow the script, to sacrifice our own well-being to meet society's expectations. In the church, my worth had been tied to my ability to be a "good wife" and uphold the ideal family unit. When I stepped outside that role, shame rushed in to try to pull me back in line. But shame isn't truth—it's just the voice of the systems that benefit from our silence and compliance.

Months later, I ended up singing in a mostly Black gospel choir in a little country church up on a hill where my parents attended. They loved my kiddo. And they loved me—a lost white woman searching for something in that church building. They didn't judge me for being single, and slowly my shame started to fade.

Shame is Useful—Until It's Not

From an evolutionary standpoint, shame served an important purpose. At one point, it helped keep clans and tribes safe—because when everyone conformed, everyone survived. If you were cast out, you wouldn't last long on your own. Shame was a built-in alarm system, warning us when our actions might lead to rejection, exile, or worse.

And that's why it still feels so powerful today.

Even though we no longer live in isolated tribes, our nervous system doesn't know that. When we feel shame, our brain treats it as a survival threat. It sends us into panic mode, convincing us we need to fix whatever we did wrong, blend in, and regain acceptance—fast.

Shame, at its core, is just trying to protect us.

Here's the problem: The world has changed, shame hasn't.

Instead of keeping us alive, it keeps us small. It convinces us that blending in is safer than standing out. It tells us that following the rules—even when those rules are outdated, oppressive, or harmful—is the only way to be accepted. It doesn't just make us cautious—it makes us afraid.

And worse? Shame is easily weaponized by others.

We see it start early. Kids shame each other on the playground for being different. They call out a classmate for stumbling in gym class or fumbling their words when the teacher calls on them. Fast forward to adulthood, and it's the same story, just with bigger consequences. Coworkers shame each other for not participating in work events, for handling projects differently, for not "playing the game" the way they think you should. At work, in social circles, even within families, shame is used to keep people in line.

Women, especially, are controlled by shame. We're shamed for being too ambitious. We're shamed for not being ambitious enough. We're shamed for wanting kids, for not wanting kids, for taking up space, for not speaking up, for speaking up too much. It's exhausting.

But here's the thing—when we feel shame, we actually have an opportunity. Instead of letting it control us, we can turn toward it. We can *talk* to it.

If you can imagine your inner landscape made up of various parts—a part that loves going to the movies, a part that gets riled up over politics, a part that feels ashamed about something, and so on—what would the part of you that's feeling ashamed want you to know? Have you ever asked?

You might be surprised at what it has to say.

Talking to Shame

How on earth do you talk to shame? The same way you'd talk to a child or teenager—gently, with curiosity and compassion. Start by going somewhere you know you won't be bothered or interrupted. Breathe deeply and imagine finding shame in your body. When you think about the thing you're feeling shame around, how does your body respond? My shame used to like to hide out in my chest, around my heart. Notice how it feels.

And then just greet it. Welcome it. Say hi to it. You might be surprised by what happens when you simply acknowledge your emotions—especially the difficult ones. They tend to open up when they feel seen.

Ask shame what information it has for you. What does it want you to know?

Often, when we ask an emotion for more insight, we realize it's really a younger part of ourselves—a part that's afraid of something. Shame is often rooted in fear: fear of being left out, unloved, unworthy. Don't take my word for it—ask your shame directly.

As you talk to this part of yourself, resist the urge to coach it, fix it, or push it away. Just hold space for it. Remind it of the beautiful things in your life. Let it know how old you are now—because often, this part of you still believes you're much younger, stuck in the moment that created the shame in the first place. And when it feels heard, shame tends to soften. Meeting it with compassion and presence is the key to releasing it.

That doesn't mean shame won't return. It will, for the same reasons or for new ones you haven't encountered yet. But when it does, it won't have the same power over you. It won't dictate your choices. Most importantly, you won't have to rely on outside validation to pull you out of it—because you'll already know how to navigate it from within.

The Shame-Burnout Connection

Shame tells us we aren't enough—so we over-perform and over-deliver, desperately trying to prove that we are. And this is where burnout happens. We make promises we can't keep. We say yes to things we don't have the time or energy for. We cancel plans at the last minute because we're too exhausted to follow through. We miss out on the world around us. And then, of course, we feel even more shame.

I've known too many women who carry shame about their body shape, their parenting skills, their job qualifications, their diet, their car, their neighborhood, their bank account— the list goes on. And why? Because the world profits from our insecurities.

How's that, you might ask? Conformity, thousands of dollars in beauty products we don't need, vacations to finally connect as a family in the midst of an over-crowded theme park (yes, Disney, I love you but wow), investments that don't pan out, "free" PDFs that come with an unhealthy helping of spammy emails, and more.

So, let me ask you something: Who actually benefits when you feel shame?

It's certainly not you, honey. It's your employer who gets an over-committer to pick up the slack for everyone else. It's the business wiz trying to sell you the "perfect" coaching package that will magically solve all your problems. (Spoiler alert: There's no one-size-fits-all coaching package.) It's the marketing machine that capitalizes on envy in the form of Snapchat filters and FOMO.

Shame just leads to more shame, more exhaustion, more overwhelm. Unless—you start talking to it *and* about it. That's how you break the cycle.

Your Highest Self Will Never Shame You

This might be the most important takeaway of this chapter: Your highest self will never shame you. Shame comes from the outside. We aren't born with it—it's taught to us. And when you start talking to shame, it's your highest self leading that conversation. Coming from this Self-energy, you can engage with the part (or parts) of you that are feeling, expressing, and reinforcing shame. And once you address it, once you bring it into the light, its grip on you weakens.

Shame holds power because it taps into one of our deepest survival instincts—the need to belong. But most of the time, we feel ashamed of things that have nothing to do with our worth. The kind of car we drive. The number in our bank account. The way our hair looks. As a kid, I carried shame about my curls, not because they were bad, but because society taught me they didn't fit the mold.

That's the thing about shame—it's about humiliation and forced assimilation.

So, remember this: YOU do not benefit from feeling ashamed. The only ones who benefit from your shame are the forces that profit from keeping you small. But even when we intellectually *know* that shame isn't ours to carry, it still helps to have people who remind us. Surrounding yourself with people who truly see and accept you can help unplug you from shame even faster.

Rely on Your Social Network Too

Shame tells us we don't belong—that we're failing in some way, that we're not measuring up. Connection reminds us that we are already enough. One of the best ways to push back against shame is to lean on the people who truly see and accept us. When we feel the weight of shame creeping in— whether it's about our bodies, our careers, our choices, or something else entirely—it helps to reach out.

Shame thrives in isolation. The more we keep it to ourselves, the stronger it gets. And when we name it out loud to the people who love us, its power starts to dissolve. A trusted friend or loved one can remind you of what's real—that you are not failing, you are not unworthy, and you are not alone.

You may be surprised to find that true belonging was there all along—you just had to reach for it.

Releasing Shame and Stress

Shame and stress go hand-in-hand. Shame can stress us out, *and* we can experience shame about our stress. So, here's a tip straight from the animal kingdom. Next time you're stressed: Shake it out.

Growing up, my dachshund, Scooter, was the world's biggest fraidy-cat. Anytime something startled him, he'd run for cover—then shake his entire body from head to tail. That shaking wasn't just random; it was his body's way of discharging stress and pent-up adrenaline. And here's the thing—our bodies need to do this too. The only difference is that we've been conditioned to "stay still and behave." To not make a scene. To keep it all inside. Well, this is your permission slip to live out loud!

The next time you're feeling stressed, literally shake it out. Find a private space—your bedroom, the shower, even a locked restroom stall at work—and shake your entire body. Start with your hands, gently roll your neck, shake your arms, wiggle your hips, bounce your knees, and yes, even shake your feet. Let everything move. It may feel silly at first, but this simple technique helps regulate your nervous system and brings you back to center.

Our bodies naturally shake when we experience extreme stress—think about how your hands tremble after a near-accident or an intense argument. That's your nervous system trying to complete the stress cycle. But in daily life, we suppress this instinct. That's why shaking intentionally is so powerful—it helps your body do what it's designed to do. And really, it's a much healthier way to release stress than some of the other techniques people use!

When my partner and I go out to eat or visit our favorite craft cocktail bar, he whips out his phone, on which he has an 84-question list of conversation-starting questions. One of the oldest on the list is, *"Would you rather be comfortable or powerful?"* Now, there's no right or wrong answer to this question. And they're also not mutually exclusive—you can be both comfortable and powerful. Yet, considering the choice between the two is the fun. Some people can't choose, but most people do.

The women who choose powerful often have big goals. They're working toward a degree. They're motivated. They've got good relationships, and they have ambition.

And by picking up this book, you've chosen to be powerful too.

Choosing to break up with burnout is uncomfortable sometimes. It means questioning things you were taught to accept. It means setting boundaries that might make people uncomfortable. It means reclaiming your time and energy in a world that profits from your exhaustion. But like all life-changing work, it's so worth it. I'm sincerely thrilled this book is in your hands. This is how we change the world—for ourselves and for the brilliant women who will follow us.

By now, I hope you can see that burnout isn't just the result of doing too much. It's the result of the narratives that drive us to overextend, overcommit, and overwork. The stories we've been told, the ones we've absorbed, and the ones we keep telling ourselves: who we're supposed to be, what we owe to others, and what it takes to be 'enough.'

But here's the thing—those stories aren't fixed. They were written by systems that weren't built for our well-being. If we want to break the cycle, we have to change the narrative.

And to do that, we have to zoom in—from the societal roots of burnout to the deeply personal ways it manifests in our lives. Because burnout isn't just theoretical—it's something you feel and experience. In your body. In your emotions. In the way you move through the world.

In Part 2, we're going deeper. We're moving from the causes of burnout to your personal experience of it. We'll explore the different types of burnout, the emotions that fuel them, and—most importantly—how to recognize your unique burnout pattern. Because once you see it clearly, you can finally start breaking free.

PART II
The Experience of Burnout

5

The Six Types of Burnout

Burnout is easy to intellectualize. It's tempting to take a high-level, academic approach—breaking it down into definitions, theories, and symptoms. But "in theory" rarely helps anyone. So let's stop talking theory and talk about how we actually experience burnout.

By now, we recognize that burnout isn't just about work. It seeps into every aspect of life—our relationships, our emotional well-being, our energy levels. Whether we've explored the research or simply felt it firsthand, we intuitively know that burnout extends beyond our jobs.

Burnout doesn't just differ in *where* it happens—it also varies in *how* it affects us. Some people feel it physically, drained of energy, no matter how much they rest. Others experience emotional exhaustion, struggling to care about things that once mattered. Some find themselves mentally overloaded, unable to process more information, while others burn out from constant social interactions.

Through my work in burnout prevention, I've identified six core types of burnout—each representing a different way it can take hold. And while we might be more vulnerable to some types than others, burnout rarely happens in isolation. Most of us experience a mix of these types at the same time.

Acute vs. Chronic Burnout

Before we dive in, it's important to understand the difference between acute and chronic burnout.

Acute burnout happens in the moment—it's temporary, often tied to a specific event or short-term stressor. Think of it as catching a cold: unpleasant, but usually recoverable with rest and care.

Chronic burnout, on the other hand, is persistent. It builds over time, flaring up repeatedly, much like chronic bronchitis. If left unaddressed, it can feel impossible to escape.

Recognizing whether your burnout is acute or chronic can help you determine the best path to recovery. Sometimes, a single day of rest can help reset your system. Other times, deeper, long-term adjustments are needed to truly break the cycle.

Which Types of Burnout Affect You Most?

Understanding which types of burnout we're most susceptible to can help us recognize our limits and make better choices about recovery. For instance, I *love* a good nap, so physical burnout isn't my biggest concern. But as someone who feels deeply for others, I know I'm highly susceptible to empathic burnout.

This next section of the book dives into each of these six burnout types—how they manifest, why they happen, and what we can do about them.

The six types of burnout are:

1. Social
2. Mental/Informational
3. Physical
4. Emotional
5. Energetic
6. Empathic

Most people will recognize themselves in more than one category—and that's normal. The key is identifying your personal burnout patterns so you can start addressing them at the root.

A Quick but Important Note

Many of the symptoms we'll discuss—exhaustion, detachment, overwhelm—can also be signs of clinical depression or anxiety.

If this feels too heavy, or if burnout has become a constant in your life, please consider reaching out to a licensed mental health professional. Burnout is real, and you don't have to navigate it alone.

Now, let's explore the six types of burnout and what they mean for you.

6

Social Burnout

Introverts, I've got you. And extroverts, you're not off the hook either—social burnout doesn't discriminate. Social burnout happens when you reach a point where being around people feels exhausting rather than energizing. You're tired of being "on," of performing, of being observed. Even social interactions you usually enjoy start to feel like obligations.

It's not just a need for alone time—it's a sign your social battery is depleted.

Social burnout means that you don't have the energy to connect with the people around you. You'll have mom guilt (funny how dad guilt isn't really a thing, huh?) and the sneaking suspicion that you're missing out on life.

Because you are.

Social burnout steals your joy for everyday interactions. Spending quality time with family, making memories with your friends, and enjoying your vacation are nearly impossible if you're wrangling social burnout. You just don't have the energy to invest in these situations and the people within them.

Signs of Social Burnout

While social burnout looks different for everyone, the following signs suggest you may be experiencing it:

- You become easily irritated by other people.
- Large groups of people stress you out when they didn't before.
- You dread the holidays when you used to love them.
- Your temper has shortened.
- You have a hard time engaging in another person's story.
- Relating to others feels harder than it used to.
- You struggle to empathize with others.

Do any of these sound familiar? Read the list again and add a little checkmark or highlight the lines that resonate with your experience. One of the biggest red flags of any form of burnout is when something that once brought you joy now drains you. If socializing used to energize you but now feels like a chore, that's burnout talking.

One of my colleagues, "Anne," recently chatted with me about her burnout experience. She's an extrovert, thrives on virtual coffee chats with people around the world, and just loves people. But after a whirlwind few weeks of launching a new product and entertaining house guests, she told me she felt completely burnt out but couldn't identify why.

So, we walked through the different types of burnout together:

- It wasn't mental burnout—she had just finished reading a book and found it inspiring.
- It wasn't emotional burnout—there was no major personal stress weighing on her.
- It wasn't physical burnout—she was getting enough sleep and staying active.
- It wasn't energetic burnout—she still felt excited about her business.
- It wasn't empathic burnout—she still cared about the people she was connecting with.

That left social burnout. She'd simply hit her limit on human interaction.

So, my recommendation to her was to unplug from social media for the rest of the day and spend intentional alone time—no Zoom calls, no texts, no social obligations. She just needed a day. She needed to retreat from the day-to-day social pressure of being "on" and from entertaining others, even though she really enjoys the social aspects of her life and work.

And wouldn't you know it? After a day to herself, she was recharged and ready to get going again. This is a great example of dealing with acute burnout, so it doesn't compound into chronic burnout. In cases of acute burnout, there's a ton of room for resolution. The chance to regroup and rest away from people was all Anne needed in order to get back on the horse again and dive right back into her launch.

Sometimes, social burnout doesn't hit all at once—it sneaks up on you. You might even mistake it for just being "a little tired" until you realize you're actively avoiding people. This is why social burnout can be so tricky to spot—especially for extroverts. It doesn't just come from not having enough alone time—it can also come from too much high-energy interaction, too quickly. You might not even realize you're burnt out until you hit a social "crash" and suddenly want to avoid everyone.

The key is learning your own patterns. If you're feeling drained, irritable, or uninterested in things you usually enjoy, your social battery might need more than a quick recharge.

Women and Social Burnout

"I'm the princess. I'm the example. I've got duties, responsibilities, expectations. My whole life is planned out." — Merida, *Brave*

As women, we're expected to be social. Not just social, but pleasant, accommodating, and available. We're taught that being likable matters, that connection is part of our role, and that withdrawing from others—even when we need to—can make us seem cold or unfriendly.

When women don't meet these expectations, we are often shamed. I know I sound like a broken record bringing up conditioning again, but social conditioning shapes every part of how we think, act, and engage with the world. It's not just about how we behave—it's about what we believe we should want, what feels acceptable, and where we feel pressured to conform. Our mothers and their mothers before them were taught that certain behaviors were appropriate and others were not. My goodness, just thinking about the things I was supposed to say and not say based on my gender as I was growing up scrambles my brain.

And it starts early. Some argue this gender conditioning begins at birth.[1] I'd argue it starts even earlier—the moment the sonographer announces "It's a girl!" From that instant, expectations start forming. Parents, grandparents, and well-meaning strangers begin making assumptions about who that child will be, how she will behave, and yes—how social she should be. Even those parents who approach their kid's earth-side existence with gender neutrality are doing so in reaction to societal norms that already exist. That's how deeply ingrained these expectations are.

And let's be honest: Girls are expected to be more social than boys. I've never once heard a boy called a *social butterfly*, but I was called one all the time growing up. If you are naturally social, that might be fine—but what if you aren't? What if

---

1. Karyn Chylewski, "Does Social Conditioning Hold Women Back from Leadership Roles?," Does Social Conditioning Hold Women Back from Leadership Roles? (BetterUp, March 10, 2021), https://www.betterup.com/blog/has-social-conditioning-been-holding-women-back-from-leadership-roles.

you feel pressure to be social even when you don't want to be?

That's when social burnout becomes even more likely.

Do Introverts Handle Social Burnout Better?

I have a theory that introverts may be better at managing social burnout than extroverts.

Since introverts naturally recharge through alone time, they tend to "practice" solitude more often. This built-in habit of stepping back might give them an edge when it comes to avoiding social burnout. In contrast, extroverts thrive on connection—which means we don't always recognize when we've overdone it.

I'll admit it: As an extrovert, I don't always know when to stop. I love people. I love conversation. I love the energy of a good gathering. But then suddenly—bam!—I hit what I call my Extrovert Limit. And when I hit it, I *really* hit it.

Because yes, even extroverts need a break from people. The difference? We're not always great at realizing when we need it.

That's why the key to avoiding social burnout is to recognize your own signs. When do *you* start feeling drained? When does social time stop feeling energizing and start feeling exhausting? Maybe it's when you no longer have patience for the beloveds in your life. Maybe it's when the mere idea of socializing makes you want to cry.

Pay attention to anticipatory anxiety—that creeping stress you feel *before* a social event even happens. Notice if large crowds start overwhelming you. And definitely watch for the ultimate red flag: when other people annoy the ever-loving hell out of you for no real reason.

These are all signals. And when you start seeing them? It's time to take a step back.

Ways to Reduce and Recover from Social Burnout

Social burnout doesn't just come from in-person interactions—it can happen virtually too. Whether it's work meetings, social media, or endless group texts, constant connection can be exhausting.

The best way to recover? Step away. It can be uncomfortable to be by ourselves, with just our inner dialogue and thoughts circling about. However, it's the best way to recover from social burnout—because you've just been around too many people!

Here are some other simple but powerful ways to recharge:

- **Put the phone down.** No scrolling. No notifications. Just give yourself a break.
- **Take a nap.** Seriously—sleep is one of the best ways to reset your nervous system.
- **Get outside.** Nature is grounding. A walk in fresh air (without your AirPods) can work wonders.
- **Lose yourself in a book.** No emails. No social feeds. Just an actual, physical book.

- **Binge a little Netflix alone** (or, you know, Netflix and chill *by yourself*... if ya know what I mean).
- **Listen to instrumental music.** Even voices in songs can feel overwhelming when you're burnt out.

The key here is to reduce your social interaction, whether that's real or perceived.

And remember: we all have different "social batteries." Some people thrive on frequent socializing, while others need more alone time to function. Honor your energy levels. Don't push yourself to be more social than you need to be.

7

Mental Burnout

"**W**hat, like it's hard?" ~ Elle Woods, *Legally Blonde.*

Yes, Elle. It's hard.

Mental burnout happens when your brain is overloaded with information, decisions, and constant input. Your mind feels like a tangled mess of open tabs—so many thoughts running at once that you can't focus on a single one. You read the same paragraph three times without absorbing a word. You forget what you walked into a room for. You feel exhausted, not from physical activity, but from the sheer effort of thinking.

In college, I had the brilliant idea to take Latin. Mainly, I did it because it's largely a written and unspoken language, so there were no oral exams that required me to stand in front of the class and try to speak a second language. I'm so glad I did it, but given the chance to do it again, I'd probably pick something like Spanish to learn for my foreign language credit. Ooh, or sign language! ASL is so cool. I digress.

Latin is exceptionally complex. To add to the complexity, the word order matters far less than the endings of the words themselves. Every noun has six forms, each changing depending on its role in the sentence. And yes—each of those also has singular and plural versions.

Take the word *Agricola* (farmer). Depending on the sentence, it could be:

- Agricola/Agricolae
- Agricolae/Agricolarum
- Agricolae/Agricolis
- Agricolam/Agricolas
- Agricola/Agricolis
- Agricola/Agricolae

Confused yet? Yep—some forms are spelled the same but mean totally different things. Oh, and don't forget grammatical gender—because everything in Latin is either masculine, feminine, or neuter, and any word modifying it has to match.

Honestly, just writing that out made my brain hurt, so I'm guessing reading it had the same effect on you. And that is exactly what mental/informational burnout feels like. It's what happens when you're absorbing too much information —whether from work, school, the news, social media, or just life—and your brain hits a wall.

Mental burnout doesn't always announce itself with a dramatic crash. It's not like physical burnout, where your body forces you to stop. Instead, mental burnout is sneaky. It builds slowly, creeping into your daily life in ways that feel normal—at least at first.

One of the reasons it's so hard to catch is that it often masquerades as productivity. You're constantly consuming information—reading articles, keeping up with industry trends, checking your email, listening to podcasts, staying "in the know." At first, it feels like you're just being diligent, staying informed, and maybe even expanding your knowledge. But over time, your brain starts to feel cluttered. You find yourself re-reading the same paragraph multiple times. You struggle to recall details. You open a tab only to forget why you opened it in the first place. What started as a commitment to learning and engagement turns into a foggy, overstuffed mental load.

Compounding this is the fact that our culture celebrates constant engagement. Being "busy" is often equated with being important, successful, or driven. Workplaces expect employees to be available, responsive, and adaptable at all times. Social media bombards us with updates, news, and endless "must-know" information. And thanks to smartphones, the line between work, personal life, and leisure is so blurred that we rarely give our brains permission to truly power down. We aren't just encouraged to keep up—we're expected to.

Mental burnout doesn't feel like exhaustion right away. Instead, it often presents as distraction, overwhelm, or indecisiveness. It actually looks a lot like ADHD. You might feel unable to concentrate for long periods, constantly jumping between tasks but finishing none of them. Decision-making —something that once felt simple—starts to feel exhausting. Even routine choices, like what to make for dinner or which emails to respond to first, become overwhelming. And because mental burnout doesn't come with the same physical symptoms as other forms of burnout, you might not realize how deep it runs until you're completely stuck— unable to focus, make decisions, or even enjoy the things that usually bring you joy.

The key to preventing mental burnout is recognizing it before it fully takes hold. That means paying attention to the early signs: Are you feeling scattered? Struggling to focus? Unable to retain information? Feeling like your brain is constantly "full"? These are signals that your mind needs a break—before it forces you to take one.

Mental burnout isn't just about feeling overwhelmed—it affects every area of life. When your brain is constantly overloaded, even small tasks feel monumental. It's like carrying a backpack that gets heavier each day. You start strong, but eventually, it wears you down and causes:

- **Decision Fatigue** – Simple choices, like what to eat for dinner, feel overwhelming.
- **Reduced Creativity & Problem-Solving** – Your brain struggles to make connections.

- **Shortened Attention Span** – You jump from task to task but can't focus.
- **Increased Anxiety & Stress** – The more information you consume, the more anxious you feel.
- **Sleep Disruptions** – Even when you're exhausted, your mind won't shut off.

If you've ever had a day where your brain just *refuses* to cooperate, where everything feels like mental quicksand, that's mental burnout at work.

Signs of Mental Burnout

Signs you may be experiencing mental burnout:

- You read the same thing multiple times and still don't absorb it.
- You struggle to focus on tasks you usually complete easily.
- You feel mentally fatigued even after resting.
- You jump between multiple tasks but struggle to finish anything.
- You procrastinate because your brain feels "too full."
- You forget important details, appointments, or tasks.
- You feel anxious, overwhelmed, or panicked about making decisions.

- You experience "brain fog" and find it harder to recall information.
- You suddenly find yourself blaming "ADHD" even if you haven't been diagnosed with it (which doesn't mean you don't have ADHD, by the way!).

Do any of these sound familiar? Take a moment to notice how your brain feels right now. If mental burnout is showing up for you, know that it's not a personal failing—it's a sign your mind needs a break.

Why do so many of us push ourselves to the point of mental burnout? One reason is that we confuse consuming with learning—just because we're constantly taking in information doesn't mean we're actually retaining or applying it. At the same time, we don't prioritize mental rest the way we do physical rest. Adding to this, we've been conditioned to believe that multitasking is a skill to master, when in reality, constantly switching between tasks makes us less productive and more susceptible to mental overload. These habits, reinforced by modern demands, keep us in a cycle of burnout without us even realizing it's happening.

Women and Mental Burnout

Women are particularly prone to mental burnout—not just because of work, but because of the mental load we carry. The invisible workload of life often falls on women's shoulders, from remembering birthdays and tracking family schedules to planning meals and managing household logistics—all on top of their professional responsibilities.

Beyond the home, there's also an unspoken expectation to stay informed on everything: current events, parenting strategies, workplace trends, and self-improvement, all at once. And then there's decision fatigue—the relentless stream of choices that need to be made daily, from major career moves to the simplest of questions, like what's for dinner. Even when we're physically still, our minds are running marathons, carrying the weight of responsibilities, expectations, and the constant pressure to keep everything running smoothly.

How Neurodivergent Folks, Creatives, And Analytical Thinkers Experience Mental Burnout Differently

Mental burnout doesn't affect everyone in the same way. Depending on how your brain is wired, the way you process information, and your personal tendencies, mental burnout might manifest differently for you than for someone else.

For neurodivergent folks (such as those with ADHD, autism, or other cognitive differences), mental burnout can be especially tricky. People with ADHD, for example, often thrive on novelty, hyper-focus, and intellectual stimulation—until they don't. The same ability to dive deep into a subject can lead to cognitive exhaustion when there's too much information to process. On the flip side, executive dysfunction—difficulty prioritizing tasks, organizing thoughts, or filtering distractions—can make mental overload feel even more chaotic. For autistic individuals, the sheer volume of sensory and informational input in daily life can lead to shutdowns, where the brain simply refuses to process more information.

This isn't laziness or avoidance—it's a neurological response to overload.

For creatives, mental burnout often sneaks in through the pressure to constantly produce. Writers, artists, designers, and musicians might find themselves hitting a creative block —not because they've lost their talent, but because their minds are simply overstimulated or they're focused more on making content than art. When your brain is in constant "input mode"—consuming news, social media, podcasts, or even other people's work—there's no space left for new ideas to emerge. Creativity requires mental white space, and when burnout clutters that space with too much information, inspiration dries up.

For analytical thinkers—those who thrive on logic, strategy, and problem-solving—mental burnout often manifests as decision fatigue and cognitive overload. People in data-heavy professions, researchers, business strategists, and planners may feel like their brains simply stop processing information effectively. Tasks that once felt stimulating now feel draining. A spreadsheet that used to make sense suddenly looks like a jumble of meaningless numbers. It's not that their intelligence has disappeared—it's that their cognitive processing power is depleted, much like a computer running too many applications at once.

Each of these groups may experience mental burnout differently, but they all share a common need: intentional mental rest. Whether it's setting boundaries around information intake, incorporating structured breaks, or allowing for unstructured, pressure-free thinking time, the solution isn't to push harder—it's to step back, reset, and give the brain time to recharge.

Ways to Reduce and Recover from Mental Burnout

The good news? Mental burnout is often easily reversible. Taking a break from your current mental load—whether it's work, studying, or life admin—can help reset your mind. But wouldn't it be even better to avoid burnout altogether?

Reduce Information Overload

Brain Dumping

Sometimes, your brain just needs a hard reset. Grab a piece of paper (or open a notes app) and write down every thought swirling in your head—tasks, worries, ideas, things to remember. Get it all out. Once it's on paper, your brain no longer has to hold it all.

Digital Detox

We absorb more information in a single day than our ancestors did in a lifetime. Social media, news updates, emails—it's too much. Set boundaries around when and how you consume information. Try turning off non-essential notifications, taking social media breaks, and setting a "news limit" (e.g., checking headlines once a day, not all day).

Work Smarter, Not Harder

Organize Your Tasks

Ever feel overwhelmed by your to-do list? That's mental burnout creeping in. Break big tasks into smaller, manageable pieces. Instead of adding "Write Book," to your to do list, break big projects down into manageable pieces with shorter term deadlines. So in my book example, I'd have a deadline for drafting the outline, another for writing the first section, and another for editing the final draft. Seeing progress in small steps makes it feel less overwhelming. Plus, when we check off more of these smaller tasks, our brains get the oh-so-important feel-good neurotransmitter, dopamine, far more often, and that keeps us moving forward..

Body Doubling

If you struggle to focus, try working alongside someone else. This technique—popular with folks with ADHD—helps with accountability and focus. Whether in-person or virtual, having someone nearby tricks your brain into staying engaged.

Pomodoro® Method

In the late 1980s, Francesco Cirillo created the Pomodoro® Method—a structured process to get stuff done. You sit down for a 25-minute work session, followed by a break that lasts for two to five minutes.[1] Then, you get back to work. It works for neurospicy and neurotypical folks, alike. In our modern

---

1. "The Pomodoro® Technique," Cirillo Company, 2023, https://francescocirillo.com/products/the-pomodoro-technique.

world, there's so much vying for our attention—we've all lost the skill of concentrated focus for longer than 20 or 30 minutes at a time. Instead of fighting your brain, work with it —use short, structured bursts to maintain focus without exhausting yourself.

Prioritize Mental Rest

Sleep Hygiene

Mental burnout gets worse when you're not sleeping well, so make sure you have sleep hygiene dialed in. You'll want to develop a simple nighttime routine to signal your brain it's time to wind down and keep a consistent sleep/wake schedule, even on weekends. Journaling before bed can help clear out mental clutter, and avoiding screens for at least an hour is important for your circadian rhythm.

Downtime Without Stimulation

If you're susceptible to mental burnout, your brain needs quiet time without input. That means no podcasts while folding laundry, no news while eating breakfast, and no scrolling social media while going to the bathroom! While I'm a big fan of meditation and mindfulness, you don't need to add another practice to your schedule. Try just sitting with your thoughts for a few minutes each day. At first, it might feel weird. But giving your brain space to rest makes a huge difference.

8

Physical Burnout

E ver felt like you just can't keep going? Like no matter how much you sleep, you wake up exhausted? That's not just being tired—that's physical burnout.

When you push your body beyond its limits—whether from lack of sleep, over-exercising, chronic stress, or simply never allowing yourself to rest—your body eventually forces you to stop. Sometimes this shows up as constant fatigue or brain fog. Other times, it's illness, headaches, stomach issues, or even a complete physical breakdown.

And yet, many of us ignore the warning signs. We assume we just need a little caffeine, a weekend to "catch up" on sleep, or a better workout routine. But physical burnout isn't just about what you do—it's about what you fail to recover from.

Like mental/informational burnout, physical burnout is pretty easy to both define and mitigate. When you've been running on fumes, your body will eventually say, "Nope.

We're done here." Sometimes this comes in the form of illness. Other times, it's just the need to sleep for 12 hours straight. And yes, some personal trainers will tell you that physical burnout only happens from maxing out your work-outs—but that's only one piece of the puzzle. Physical burnout doesn't just come from over-exercising—it also comes from under-recovery.

Signs of Physical Burnout

One of the biggest signs that I'm physically burned out is that I start feeling really run down. I may even run a little low-grade fever until I sleep it off. Since we all have different relationships with our bodies, physical burnout can have a wide variety of symptoms. Physical burnout may look like:

- **Brain fog** struggling to think clearly or focus.
- **GI issues** – stomach upset, diarrhea, nausea... all the unpleasant stuff.
- **Headaches** that just won't quit.
- **Insomnia** – yes, seriously. Burning out can make it **harder** to sleep, not easier.
- **Low sex drive** – your body is too drained to care.
- **Struggles with basic self-care** – even brushing your teeth can feel like a chore.
- **Second-guessing yourself** – burnout makes decision-making feel impossible.

One of the most fascinating (and frustrating) things about physical burnout is that it messes with our confidence. When our bodies are run down, our minds follow. We start doubting ourselves, questioning every little decision—even ones we wouldn't think twice about normally.

That's because burnout isn't just physical—it's a full-body, mind-body experience.

Let's Talk About the Mind-Body Relationship

I don't remember exactly when I became aware of the deep connection between my mind and body. At this point, it feels like I've always understood it—but I know that's not true.

In my early 30s, I became a certified meditation teacher in a modality called Neurosculpting®, which blends neuro-science with traditional guided meditation to strengthen the link between the body and the mind. Although I'm no longer part of the Neurosculpting Institute (NSI), the knowledge I gained there stays with me today. Through this practice, I learned to tune into my body—to actually feel where emotions and energy were stored.

That experience opened the door to other modalities, including The Emotion Code, which suggests that we physi-cally store emotions in our bodies. While I don't align with everything taught in The Emotion Code, this fundamental idea makes a lot of sense to me.

You've probably felt butterflies in your stomach before a big moment. That's not just a saying—it's because we actually have neurons (a.k.a. brain cells) in our gut, too. If this is new information to you, you're probably having the same mind-blown reaction I did when I first learned about it. Our bodies are a vast neural network that extends from our brain through every system—so, of course, our mental and physical states are deeply intertwined.

It reminds me of poor Luisa in *Encanto*. When the magic at the Casita starts failing, Luisa is the first to feel it. *"Mirabel and I were having this little talk about me carrying too much, so I tried not to carry so much, but I realized it was putting me behind, and I knew I was gonna let everyone down and I felt really bad,"* she says in one breath when Abuela asks what's wrong. *"But when I went to throw the donkeys in the barn, they were...heavy!"* She wails and runs away. She's clearly carrying too much—both metaphorically and literally!

The same thing happens to us. When we're mentally exhausted, we feel the physical effects—like the urge to collapse into a nap. And when we push ourselves too hard physically, our mental health takes a hit. That's why caring for both your mind and body daily isn't just a nice idea—it's essential.

Women and Physical Burnout

Women are uniquely vulnerable to physical burnout, not just because of demanding schedules, but due to biological and systemic factors that make true recovery more challenging. Chronic sleep deprivation is a major contributor, as studies consistently show that women—especially working mothers—get less sleep than men. Hormonal fluctuations throughout the menstrual cycle, pregnancy, perimenopause, and menopause can further disrupt sleep quality, leaving many women in a near-constant state of fatigue that compounds over time.

Beyond sleep, medical gaslighting plays a significant role in why women experience physical burnout more acutely. Women's pain, exhaustion, and symptoms of chronic illness are more likely to be dismissed by healthcare providers, often being written off as stress, anxiety, or simply "normal" female experiences. This leads to delays in diagnosis and treatment, forcing many women to push through genuine physical distress without the medical support they need. When your symptoms are repeatedly ignored or minimized, you internalize the message that you're supposed to just "handle it"—which only accelerates burnout.

Additionally, women are disproportionately affected by chronic illnesses and autoimmune diseases, which can make physical burnout an unavoidable reality. Conditions like fibromyalgia, lupus, Hashimoto's thyroiditis, and chronic fatigue syndrome are all more prevalent in women, yet they remain widely misunderstood and often under-researched. Living with these conditions means navigating persistent fatigue, muscle pain, and brain fog—on top of daily responsibilities. And because these illnesses often have invisible symptoms, many women feel pressured to function at full capacity even when their bodies are signaling the opposite.

For women, physical burnout is rarely just about needing a nap—it's about recognizing that deeper, systemic neglect makes us disproportionately susceptible to this type of burnout. And while physical burnout can be acute, in women, it is far more likely to be experienced in its chronic form.

Chronic Physical Burnout from Injury or Illness

While acute physical burnout can be resolved with rest and recovery, chronic physical burnout is a different beast altogether. This type of burnout develops over time, often due to long-term injury, chronic pain, or illness, leaving you in a constant state of exhaustion that doesn't simply disappear with a nap or a weekend off.

When your body is always in distress, whether from an injury that never fully heals or an illness that flares up unpredictably, exhaustion becomes a way of life. A friend of mine lived with a severe back injury for years, and no matter how much physical therapy, medication, or rest she built into her routine, she was always drained. The sheer effort of existing in pain wore her down in ways she never anticipated —mentally, emotionally, and socially, not just physically.

Likewise, if you live with an autoimmune disease, a neurological disorder, or another chronic condition, you know the weight of physical burnout all too well. Many of these conditions come with unpredictable symptoms—fatigue that hits like a freight train, inflammation that makes movement unbearable, or brain fog that scrambles even simple tasks. And because these conditions often fluctuate, it can feel impossible to plan for recovery.

This is what makes chronic physical burnout particularly insidious—it's not something you can always bounce back from with time off or a little extra sleep. Instead, it requires an entirely different approach, one that prioritizes sustainable energy management over temporary fixes. It also demands an awareness of the emotional toll that comes with living in a body that feels like it's working against you. Because when you're constantly dealing with pain or fatigue, it doesn't just drain your physical strength —it chips away at your motivation, resilience, and mental well-being.

While there's no one-size-fits-all solution, the following strategies can help reduce the impact of chronic physical burnout. These won't eliminate the root cause of your exhaustion, but they can help you reclaim small pockets of energy, build resilience, and prevent complete depletion. If you're struggling to manage ongoing physical burnout, I strongly encourage you to seek support from a doctor, therapist, coach, or specialist who can help you navigate both the physical and emotional challenges of long-term burnout.

Ways to Reduce and Recover from Physical Burnout

Prioritize Real Rest (Not Just Sleep)

Sleep is essential, but rest and recovery go beyond just logging eight hours.

- Physical rest: Massage, stretching, or just putting your feet up.
- Sensory rest: Unplug from screens, bright lights, and noise.

- Emotional rest: Give yourself permission to *not* be productive.
- Social rest: Take space away from energy-draining interactions.

When your body signals exhaustion, listen. Overriding it with caffeine or "pushing through" doesn't make you stronger—it makes burnout worse. For more on the different types of rest, flip ahead to Chapter 21.

Rebuild Your Energy Reserves

Your body needs fuel to recover. If you're not eating enough, not drinking enough water, or running on stress hormones, your body stays stuck in burnout mode.

- Hydrate. (Seriously. Drink some water.)
- Eat nutrient-dense foods that actually support your body.
- Prioritize movement that feels good, not punishing.

Schedule Body Care (Before You Crash)

If you benefit from bodywork like massage, Reiki, chiropractic care, or acupuncture, schedule it on your calendar before you hit a burnout wall. Personally, I experience the world through my body in such a big way that I can't go without a monthly massage and chiropractic appointment. There's something deeply soothing and healing about being cared for by someone else—especially another woman. I know I'm fortunate to be able to do this, and I also recognize that not everyone has access to these services. If something like a massage isn't in your budget, look into community yoga or meditation classes. Even a simple, guided relaxation session can work wonders for helping your body unwind.

Pay Attention to Persistent Fatigue

If you've adjusted your schedule, prioritized recovery, and still feel physically drained, it's time to check in with a doctor. Hormonal imbalances, thyroid issues, and autoimmune conditions can all masquerade as burnout—but they won't improve without proper care. If your exhaustion feels chronic, it's not just in your head. Advocate for yourself. If traditional doctors are gaslighting you, consider alternative practitioners or seek a second (or third) opinion.

9

Emotional Burnout

Emotional burnout hits when you've reached your absolute emotional breaking point. It's like hitting a wall—not just physically, but mentally and emotionally, too. While emotional exhaustion is already a core symptom of burnout, emotional burnout takes it into overdrive.

When we're experiencing prolonged stress, our emotions become raw, frayed, and unmanageable. We start feeling like we're one big, exposed nerve walking around—every little thing grating against us. And unfortunately, it's not the socially acceptable emotions that get amplified, but the ones we're often taught to suppress:

- **Anger** that bubbles up at the smallest inconveniences.
- **Anxiety** that makes even simple tasks feel overwhelming.

- **Restlessness** that keeps you tossing and turning at night.
- **Sadness** that lingers, even when nothing is "wrong."
- **Irritability** that makes even casual conversations exhausting.

When emotional burnout sets in, it feels like you have nothing left to give. You're drained, reactive, and constantly teetering on the edge of frustration or overwhelm.

A prolonged sense of out-of-control emotions is a surefire way to tell that you're in the thick of emotional burnout. But it doesn't always feel like intense distress—it can also feel like you're completely tapped out.

Some of the most emotionally exhausting moments in life happen during major transitions—divorce, the death of a loved one, having a new baby, planning a wedding, buying a house. Even positive life events can be emotionally depleting. The emotional highs and stress of these experiences trigger spikes of adrenaline, causing faster breathing, sweating, and elevated heart rates—all physical symptoms of the fight-flight-freeze-or-fawn response.

This constant state of heightened emotional arousal takes a toll. Over time, we build up cortisol, which weakens the immune system, disrupts sleep, and increases vulnerability to full-blown burnout. You may feel on edge all the time, snapping at loved ones, avoiding social interactions, or feeling completely disengaged from things that once brought you joy.

Signs of Emotional Burnout

Emotional burnout affects both the body and the mind. Some of the most common symptoms include:

- **Physical Symptoms:**
  - Headaches
  - Muscle tension or soreness
  - Changes in appetite (overeating or loss of appetite)
  - Fatigue or difficulty sleeping
- **Cognitive & Emotional Symptoms:**
  - Forgetfulness
  - Difficulty concentrating
  - Apathy or feeling emotionally numb
  - Helplessness, like nothing you do makes a difference
  - Increased social anxiety
  - Feeling like a failure or "not enough"
  - A complete lack of creativity, imagination, or enthusiasm

Many of these symptoms overlap with anxiety and depression, which is why emotional burnout can sometimes go unnoticed until it reaches a breaking point. If you see yourself in this list, it's time to take a step back and prioritize emotional recovery.[1]

---

1. Erin Eatough, "22 Ways to Treat and Navigate Emotional Exhaustion," 22 Ways to Treat and Navigate Emotional Exhaustion, June 1, 2021, https://www.betterup.com/blog/emotional-exhaustion.

Women and Emotional Burnout

Women are especially vulnerable to emotional burnout due to a lifetime of conditioning that encourages emotional labor without emotional support. From a young age, many of us are taught to prioritize others' feelings over our own. We're told to be accommodating, to keep the peace, and to absorb the emotions of those around us. This expectation of constant emotional availability is exhausting—and over time, it leads to burnout.

Sometimes, it feels like women have very few emotionally safe spaces. We carry the emotional burden in our relationships and households, often serving as the default listener, mediator, and problem-solver for our families. In professional settings, we're expected to soothe tensions, "soften" direct feedback, and maintain a friendly, approachable demeanor—whether we feel like it or not. And even in society at large, we are constantly bombarded with messages telling us to be nice, to smile more, and to prioritize everyone else's comfort—even at the expense of our own well-being.

Emotional burnout happens when we've given too much for too long without replenishing ourselves. And when we do try to pull back, we're often met with guilt. We're so used to over-giving that even the idea of saying "no" feels uncomfortable.

This is why learning to set emotional boundaries is one of the most important skills for avoiding emotional burnout.

Who's Most at Risk?

People who give beyond their emotional capacity—such as caregivers, teachers, and medical professionals—are at the highest risk of emotional burnout.

Caregivers of aging parents, sick loved ones, or children with special needs often have little time to process their own emotions because they are constantly attending to someone else's needs.

Teachers face mounting pressure, shrinking resources, and, in many states, a constant fight for respect, proper pay, and basic work-life balance.

Healthcare and emergency workers (ER staff, paramedics, physicians, social workers) absorb high levels of trauma every day. When the demands never let up, emotional resilience starts to wear thin.

However, emotional burnout isn't limited to certain professions. Anyone who regularly suppresses their own emotions, overextends their emotional energy, or feels trapped in emotionally taxing relationships can experience this type of burnout. (I'm looking at you, people-pleasers and perfectionists.) Over time, without proper boundaries and recovery strategies, these personality traits and tendencies can make emotional burnout an ongoing cycle, rather than an occasional challenge.

Ways to Reduce and Recover from Emotional Burnout

One of the biggest challenges in recovering from emotional burnout is finding time for yourself. When you're constantly doing all the things, all the time, for all the people in your life, carving out personal space can feel impossible. But even small changes can make a world of difference. In addition to the strategies below, if emotional burnout is one of your types, be sure to read Chapter 18 for a primer on boundary setting.

Start With These Three Non-Negotiables

- **30 minutes of uninterrupted time to yourself every day.** No phone, no kids, no distractions—just you. A quiet morning walk, journaling, or simply sitting in stillness can reset your emotional state.
- **A consistent sleep schedule.** Getting seven to nine hours of sleep each night and going to bed and waking up at the same time every day (even on weekends!) helps regulate your mood and stress levels. Fun fact: Women biologically require more sleep than men, so getting somewhere near 10 hours of sleep each night might be your sweet spot.
- **Intentional breaks from emotional labor.** If you spend all day supporting others, take moments where you don't have to hold space for anyone else—whether it's by turning off

notifications, declining a phone call, or simply choosing not to engage in draining conversations.

Lean on a Support System That Doesn't Drain You

Having a solid support system is crucial—but make sure you're surrounding yourself with people who don't demand more emotional labor from you. The goal is to be supported, not further depleted.

Dolly Parton's Truvy in *Steel Magnolias* put it best: *"I have a strict policy that nobody cries alone in my presence."*

That's the kind of safe, supportive presence you need when you're emotionally burnt out—not someone who drains you further.

If you notice that certain relationships leave you feeling exhausted rather than supported, it's worth evaluating how much energy you're investing in them.

10

Energetic Burnout

E nergetic burnout is one of the most misunderstood forms of burnout—mainly because we don't talk about energy management the same way we talk about physical, emotional, or mental health.

Imagine sitting in a circle of 50 women, tables arranged in a horseshoe formation. Each woman is exploring the darker parts of herself—admitting fears and saying goodbye to old stories that used to govern their lives. One person speaks at a time, while everyone else holds space for her. The air is thick with emotion, vulnerability, and transformation.

If just reading that makes you want to take a deep breath and put this book down—welcome to the Energetic Burnout Club.

I love retreats. And yet, every time I attend one, I need days to recover afterward.

Energetic burnout is what happens when we absorb too much energy from the people, spaces, and emotions around us. If you consider yourself an empath, healer, or deeply intuitive person, you've likely felt this before. We're all connected energetically, but some of us are more sensitive to those connections than others. When we engage deeply with other people—whether in social settings, work environments, or healing spaces—our energetic reserves deplete.

Energetic burnout is different from emotional burnout (which comes from personal stress and deep emotional strain) and social burnout (which happens when we're over-stimulated by people). Instead, energetic burnout is about what we absorb, even when we're not actively engaging. It happens after big social events, transformational experiences, or even long periods of holding space for others.

Signs of Energetic Burnout

Energetic burnout manifests as a deep depletion—not just physically, but on an almost soul level. You may experience:

- **Apathy** – A loss of emotional connection, even to things you care about.
- **Fatigue** – A bone-deep exhaustion that sleep doesn't fix.
- **Disconnection from people** – Even loved ones may feel like "too much" right now.
- **Lack of focus** – Struggling with decision-making or deep thinking.

- **Feeling misaligned** – A vague sense that your energy is "off," but you're not sure why.

You might hit an energetic wall even after something positive —a weekend retreat, a high-energy vacation, or an exhilarating work event. You enjoyed it, but you still feel drained by it.

That's exactly what happened to a friend of mine after performing in a shadow cast production of *The Rocky Horror Picture Show*. If you've seen it performed live, you know it's a roaring good time, with energetic dance scenes, call-outs from the audience, props, and usually late-night showings. If you haven't experienced this yet, you should—as long as you're ok with some R-rated shenanigans. It's a blast—but it's also a lot.

My friend thought they were having the time of their life. But after the final performance, they hit a wall.

They weren't just physically exhausted from late-night rehearsals and sore feet. They were completely energetically drained. For days, they found themselves avoiding text messages, dodging invitations, and feeling irrationally annoyed by even small social interactions.

It took them two full weeks to want to go out again—even to their favorite '70s dance bar, where they normally thrived.

This is key: You can love an experience and still get burned out from it. If you pour out more energy than you have in reserves, you'll have nothing left for yourself.

Women and Energetic Burnout

Women are particularly susceptible to energetic burnout because we are often conditioned to be attuned to the needs, emotions, and unspoken energies of those around us. From a young age, many women are encouraged to be emotionally receptive, intuitive, and accommodating, making us more likely to absorb the energetic weight of situations without even realizing it.

But energetic burnout isn't just about taking on other people's emotions—it's about expending energy in ways that leave us depleted, even when the experience itself was positive. Women often take on the role of the emotional anchor in social, professional, and family settings, leading conversations, holding space, and managing the subtle dynamics of group interactions. Whether it's facilitating connection at a work event, attending an intensive workshop, or even hosting a family gathering, we invest unseen energy in creating harmony and ensuring others feel comfortable.

This output leaves little room for our own energetic restoration, making it difficult to discern what is truly ours and what we've absorbed from others. And because we are taught to prioritize relationships and engagement, many women struggle to recognize the need for reintegration after an energetically demanding event—often jumping back into responsibilities before fully replenishing their reserves. Understanding this pattern is key to breaking the cycle and giving ourselves permission to recover before we hit a complete energetic crash.

Going Beyond Sensitivity

While anyone can experience energetic burnout, certain groups are more prone to absorbing and carrying external energy—sometimes without realizing it. This isn't just about being naturally "sensitive." It's about the ways different people are conditioned, wired, or placed in environments that make them more susceptible to energetic overload.

Highly Intuitive & Perceptive People

If you naturally pick up on the unspoken—a shift in someone's tone, the tension in a room, or the emotional undercurrent of a conversation—you're more likely to experience energetic burnout. The more perceptive you are, the more energy you unconsciously take in. Over time, this can become mentally and physically exhausting, leaving you feeling disconnected from your own needs and emotions.

People in Leadership, Facilitator & Service Roles

If your job or lifestyle requires you to hold space for others, make decisions, or maintain an aura of calm, you may be absorbing more energy than you realize. Leaders, managers, coaches, and service-based entrepreneurs often find themselves acting as emotional anchors for others, constantly holding and managing energy in a way that leaves little room for their own processing.

People Who Work in High-Energy Environments

Those in fast-paced, high-intensity jobs—such as event planners, hospitality workers, emergency responders, or entertainers—are exposed to large amounts of external energy on a regular basis. Even when the energy is positive, the sheer volume of interactions can leave them feeling drained, overstimulated, or disconnected from themselves.

Those Who Struggle with Boundaries

If you have trouble saying no, protecting your time, or distinguishing your emotions from others, energetic burnout can hit even harder. Without clear energetic boundaries, you may find yourself constantly picking up on and carrying the stress, emotions, and expectations of those around you—often at the expense of your own well-being.

Understanding how energetic burnout manifests differently in different people is the first step to recognizing it in yourself. If you find yourself constantly feeling drained, overstimulated, or disconnected after certain interactions or environments, it may be time to start protecting your energy more intentionally.

Ways to Reduce and Recover from Energetic Burnout

Reintegration Periods

In our productivity-obsessed culture, we're expected to get right back to work after big events, experiences, or vacations.

But you need space to process, ground yourself, and recover before re-entering daily life.

I call it a reintegration period. And it is simple: Give yourself an extra day before jumping back into responsibilities. If you're coming back from vacation or time away from work, don't immediately check emails or texts and, if you can, take a full day or two on the backend of your vacation to ease back into normal life. If you're coming off a big event, work related or otherwise, avoid scheduling big projects or meetings for a day or two.

Daily Energetic Hygiene

If you experience energetic burnout, you'll want to start implementing some basic energetic hygiene practices. These are easy to do and designed to integrate into your daily life. Like brushing your teeth or taking a shower are basics for your physical body, your energetic body has some basic maintenance needs as well.

- **Ground yourself daily.** Walk barefoot outside, meditate, or do breathwork.
- **Take energetic "showers."** Imagine washing away the emotions and energy of others at the end of the day. Or actually hop in the shower and clean your physical body while cleansing your energetic body.

- **Wear protective energy colors.** Some people find wearing black, deep blue, or grounding earth tones helps shield them from absorbing external energy.
- **Create an "off-limits" day.** Set a day where you don't schedule anything and let yourself recharge however you need.
- **Connect with *yourself* before reconnecting with others.** Journal, stretch, nap—whatever feels right for your energy levels.

11

Empathic Burnout

E mpathic burnout is what happens when caring becomes overwhelming. Unlike emotional burnout, which is rooted in your own emotions, or energetic burnout, which stems from absorbing external energy, empathic burnout happens when you take on the emotional burdens of others—so much so that you have nothing left to give.

During the pandemic, a dear friend of mine—a healthcare worker—confessed something she never thought she'd say out loud: she was struggling to care.

Day after day, she treated patients who had done everything right—worn masks, gotten vaccinated, taken precautions— and still ended up critically ill. And yet, there were people running around ignoring every precaution, caught up in political debates rather than public health. It became harder for her to empathize with those who refused to protect themselves and others.

She wasn't alone.

We all have limits to how much we can hold for others. Even when we deeply care about the people in our lives, our hearts and souls have a threshold.

In the first *Wonder Woman* movie, Diana fights Ares, the god of war. When he tells her that humans don't deserve protection, she delivers this powerful statement: *"It's not about 'deserve,' it's about what you believe. And I believe in love."* Love makes us do powerful things, say yes to things we wouldn't normally say yes to, and sacrifice ourselves for the sake of others. And while that's beautiful, it also has limits.

Empathic burnout happens when we reach the point where we can no longer emotionally engage with the suffering of others. It's not that we don't want to care—it's that we're completely depleted. If you have a chronic illness, you may have experienced this firsthand. Someone complains about a minor cold and, instead of empathy, your first thought is: *Must be nice for that to be your biggest problem.* I've been there. It's not that you don't care—it's that you're totally spent.

And in today's world, there's no shortage of reasons to feel drained.

We're constantly exposed to news of injustice, suffering, and global crises. The fight for women's rights, racial justice, and human dignity is an ongoing battle. Add in natural disasters, wars, and personal struggles—and it's no wonder we're exhausted.

Signs of Empathic Burnout

Empathic burnout often begins subtly, creeping in as empathy fatigue—that feeling of being emotionally drained, detached, or overwhelmed by the suffering of others. At first, you might just feel a little exhausted—but over time, it can become a full-blown shutdown.

Empathic burnout can look like:

- **Withdrawing from others** – even people you love
- **Feeling disconnected** from the world around you
- **Exhaustion that rest doesn't fix** – you wake up just as tired as when you went to bed
- **Apathy toward causes, people, or responsibilities** you once cared deeply about
- **A sense of helplessness** – like nothing you do will make a difference
- **Overwhelm** – the weight of everything feels too heavy
- **Mood swings** – anger, sadness, frustration, or even depression
- **Self-blame** – feeling guilty for not caring "enough"[1]

---

1. "Empathy Fatigue: How It Takes a Toll on You," Cleveland Clinic (Cleveland Clinic, August 29, 2021), https://health.clevelandclinic.org/empathy-fatigue-how-stress-and-trauma-can-take-a-toll-on-you/.

Physical symptoms include trouble concentrating, headaches, nausea, conflicts in relationships, racing thoughts, insomnia[2], and all the other symptoms you've likely come to expect from burnout while reading this book.

Women and Empathic Burnout

Women are uniquely vulnerable to empathic burnout—not just because we care, but because we're expected to care. Deeply. Constantly. And often at our own expense. We've already touched on how women are cast as default caretakers, emotional laborers, and space-holders, but empathic burnout in women is fueled by something even deeper: the weight of systemic inequality and injustice that we hold in addition to our personal struggles.

We often experience systemic inequality, discrimination, and societal pressures in a way that men do not. From the fight for reproductive rights to the gender wage gap, the sheer awareness of how much work still needs to be done can create a sense of overwhelming fatigue and despair. The expectation that women must always be compassionate, patient, and endlessly understanding, even in the face of harm, discrimination, or outright oppression, leaves many of us drained.

For many women, burnout doesn't just come from caring, but from not knowing where to draw the line. How do we stay engaged without absorbing all the suffering? Where do we place our boundaries so that our empathy remains a

---

2. Ibid.

strength, not a source of depletion? Learning how to protect our energy without disconnecting from the world is one of the biggest challenges women face when navigating empathic burnout.

How Different Personality Types Experience Empathic Burnout

Empathic burnout doesn't affect everyone in the same way. Depending on your temperament, sensitivities, and how you engage with others emotionally, the way you process and experience empathic exhaustion can vary greatly.

Highly Sensitive People

Highly sensitive people (HSPs) naturally absorb the emotions of those around them. They're the ones who cry during commercials, sense shifts in a friend's mood before anything is said, and feel emotionally raw after witnessing injustice or suffering. Because they have a heightened emotional awareness, they tend to take on others' struggles as if they were their own, making them more susceptible to burnout. For HSPs, empathic burnout often feels like an overwhelming emotional flood, leaving them drained, over-stimulated, and desperate for solitude to regulate their emotions.

Therapists, Coaches, & Emotional Caretakers

People who work in helping professions—therapists, life coaches, counselors, social workers—often experience a slow, creeping onset of empathic burnout. At first, they may feel deeply connected to their clients, invested in their growth, and energized by their work. But over time, the cumulative weight of holding space for others can become emotionally unsustainable. They might start feeling emotionally detached, impatient, or even cynical about the work they once loved—signs that their emotional reserves are running dangerously low.

Activists, Advocates, & Social Justice Warriors

For those engaged in activism and advocacy, empathic burnout can feel like a deep, existential exhaustion. Fighting systemic oppression, advocating for change, and constantly confronting injustice can make it seem like no amount of effort will ever be enough. The cycle of witnessing suffering, pushing for change, and meeting resistance can lead to despair, numbness, and a sense of futility. Instead of feeling angry or motivated, they might start feeling disconnected from the very causes that once fueled them.

Logical, Analytical, & Solution-Oriented Thinkers

For those who approach the world through logic and problem-solving, empathic burnout can feel uniquely frustrating. Instead of being emotionally overwhelmed, they may feel helpless and ineffective—unable to fix what's broken or change the suffering they see around them. This type of burnout often presents as intellectual exhaustion, apathy, or avoidance rather than emotional overwhelm. They might disengage entirely, dismissing emotional issues as unsolvable or "not my problem," not out of a lack of compassion, but as a protective mechanism.

Each of these groups may experience empathic burnout in different ways, but the common thread is this: caring without boundaries leads to depletion. The key isn't to stop caring—it's to learn how to protect and replenish your emotional reserves so that you can continue showing up for others without losing yourself in the process.

Ways to Reduce and Recover from Empathic Burnout

So, how do we protect ourselves from empathy fatigue—or recover from empathic burnout when it's already set in? Susan Albers, PsyD, has a great tool. Dr. Albers calls it the ABC model: Awareness, Balance, and Connection.[3]

Awareness

The first step is recognizing when you've hit your limit. Pay attention to your emotions. If you find yourself feeling numb, detached, or easily irritated, it's time to take a step back. Instead of pushing through, practice self-compassion. Remind yourself that you are not responsible for carrying the world's pain alone.

---

3. Ibid.

Balance

I'll be honest—I'm not a huge fan of the word "balance." It's often thrown around in conversations about work/life balance (which, let's be real, is a myth). But in this model, balance is less about perfect equilibrium and more about managing your energy. Empathic burnout often happens because we give too much without refilling our own emotional cup. Finding balance doesn't mean caring less—it means caring smarter. So limit your exposure to distressing news and social media, set emotional boundaries (you can support others without absorbing their emotions), and give yourself permission to disconnect or take a break.

Think of it like an oxygen mask on a plane—you can't help others if you're running on empty.

Connection

Not all connection is draining. Spending time with people who uplift, inspire, and energize you can help counteract the effects of empathic burnout. So prioritize one-on-one time with close friends, engage in lighthearted activities (laughter is a great emotional reset), and remember that sometimes we really just need to connect back to *ourselves*. The key is to seek out relationships that pour back into you, rather than those that demand more from you.

12

The Emotions of Burnout

Burnout doesn't always announce itself with exhaustion. Sometimes, it sneaks in through irritation —snapping at your partner over something small. Or through guilt—feeling like you *should* be grateful when, really, you're just overwhelmed. Maybe it shows up as resentment— watching a coworker set a boundary you're too afraid to claim for yourself. Or it might even disguise itself as excitement—throwing yourself into a new project with so much enthusiasm that you don't notice the warning signs of overextension until it's too late.

Our emotions are not just symptoms of burnout, they're also signals. They tell us when something is unsustainable, when we're overextended, and when we're out of alignment with what we truly want. But too often, we dismiss them. We push through frustration, silence our resentment, and ignore that quiet voice inside us that says: *this isn't working.*

To break up with burnout, we have to understand the role our emotions play. And to do that, we need to step back and examine how we've been taught to experience and express emotions in the first place.

From the womb, we're judged by our behavior. Parents start making guesses about a baby's temperament based on how much they kick or wiggle around in utero. And when we pop out, we're a "good" baby or a "hard" baby, based on how well we eat, sleep, and "behave." I put the word behave in quotation marks because I don't really believe that babies behave. They react. Babies are helpless, after all, and the only parts of their brains that are fully formed are the parts that ensure survival. A baby isn't misbehaving because they're crying. They're crying because they're hungry/wet/tired/cold/scared. It's a reaction. Yet, just as we anthropomorphize our pets, we impress our values and understanding on our babies.

As we grow up, we begin learning what it means to be "good" or "bad." (Again, I use quotation marks because good and bad are subjective and socially defined rather than intrinsic.) What's deemed *good* is what makes other people comfortable, and what's deemed *bad* is often what disrupts or challenges expectations. Some emotions, like sadness or fear, might be met with comfort—while others, like anger or frustration, are met with discomfort or even punishment.

This social conditioning doesn't just shape our behavior—it shapes our burnout. If you've ever felt guilty for resting, ashamed for setting a boundary, or resentful for carrying an invisible emotional workload, you're not alone. Our relationship with burnout is deeply intertwined with the stories we've been told about which emotions are acceptable and which ones aren't.

We've already seen the stark role shame plays in fueling burnout, and in this chapter, we'll explore how other emotions play a role in the cycle, why some emotions—like anger, anxiety, and resentment—tend to hit hardest, and how learning to recognize and validate your emotions is the first step toward breaking free from burnout's grip.

Anger

As women, we're taught that anger is unacceptable. If we express it, we risk being seen as difficult, dramatic, or "too much." And because of that conditioning, we often judge ourselves just as harshly as others do.

The truth is that no emotion is inherently bad. Emotions just are. And anger? It's one of the most informative emotions we have. But when we ignore it, repress it, or try to "be nice" instead, it festers, and that's when burnout creeps in.

Anger tells us when a boundary has been crossed that we didn't realize we needed to establish. When we don't listen, we overextend ourselves. If you feel irritated every time someone interrupts you, that's a sign that your time and presence aren't being respected. If you don't acknowledge that frustration and set a boundary, you'll keep saying "yes" when you want to say "no" until you hit a breaking point.

Anger tells us when we're carrying too much. It's not just an emotion, it's a warning system. If you're constantly angry at work, at home, or in your relationships, it might not be because you're a short-tempered person—it might be because you're exhausted and running on empty.

Anger also tells us where there's sadness and regret. It's one of the stages of grief, after all. We get angry when we can't fix what's been lost, when regret feels unbearable, when we feel powerless. In those moments, we lash out, not because we're "bad" or "wrong," but because we're trying to feel something other than pain.

The only way through anger is through it. Pushing it down won't make it disappear—it'll just show up somewhere else, often disguised as resentment, exhaustion, or even self-doubt. The energy it takes to suppress anger is staggering. We put on a smile, say "It's fine," and push through. But emotional labor is labor, and if we're constantly swallowing our feelings, we're doing double the work. That's a direct road to burnout.

When anger rises, pause and ask yourself: What is this trying to tell me?

I get angry at social injustice, when someone is victimized, and when I'm disrespected. Even if you knew nothing else about me, you'd already have a pretty good idea of what I value, just by knowing what triggers my anger.

So, what about you?

Most people I know get angry when they witness cruelty. If you value compassion, then selfish, unkind behavior might make your blood boil. If you value intelligence, then seeing someone mocked for being smart might enrage you.

Your anger isn't the problem. Ignoring it is. When we listen to anger, we can set better boundaries, protect our energy, and prevent burnout before it takes over.

Anxiety

Anxiety can show up in myriad ways, but one thing's for sure: when you're burned out, your anxiety will rise. Sounds are louder. Fabric feels scratchier. Annoyances that once barely registered now feel unbearable. This heightened sensitivity is a direct result of burnout. When your nervous system is overloaded, even the smallest stressors feel amplified.

Anxiety is also one of burnout's biggest accelerators. The more exhausted you are, the harder it becomes to regulate your emotions. When you're running on empty, your brain goes into survival mode, scanning for threats—whether that's an upcoming deadline, an awkward conversation, or just the feeling that you're falling behind. And when you don't have the energy to process those worries rationally, anxiety takes over.

According to the Anxiety & Depression Association of America, over 40 million adults experience an anxiety disorder each year, with countless more struggling with everyday anxiety. The World Health Organization reports that 1 in 13 people around the globe suffer from anxiety.[1] However, just because you experience anxiety doesn't mean

---

1. "What Is Anxiety?," What Is Anxiety, 2021, https://whatisanxiety. adaa.org/.

you have an anxiety disorder. (Again, seek the help of a licensed professional if you think you might have an anxiety disorder.)

Everyday anxiety is completely normal. It's the worry over bills, the nervous energy before a big presentation, or the momentary panic when your phone battery dies and you're waiting for an important call. Everyday anxiety can also include fear of a dangerous situation or object.[2] It reminds me of a *Family Guy* episode in which Peter Griffin tells the Cowardly Lion from *The Wizard of Oz* that he's not paranoid—the flying monkeys are really scary! Everyday anxiety is real. Just because it's not a disorder doesn't mean it can't cause you issues. When everyday anxiety becomes chronic, it wears you down and that's when it starts to fuel burnout.

The thing about anxiety is this: It's not about the present moment. When we experience anxiety, we're thinking about something that happened in the past or something that might happen in the future. We're not thinking about the right now. Have you ever thought back to a terribly embarrassing moment in middle school? I have a few memories that used to make me feel the stress and embarrassment all over again when I thought about them years later. They're those ultimate cringe moments that we wish we could just erase from our mental memory banks.

Here's the thing, when something happens in the past, we can't change it. If we've harmed someone, we can go back and try to fix it. We can't erase it. What we can do is decide

---

2. Ibid.

to call it done and move on with our life. In Part 3, I give you a Time Stamp exercise to try that's designed to do this very thing!

And not to sound cliché, but no one thinks about what you were doing in middle school anymore. They probably have their own retrospective embarrassment to worry about!

So that covers the anxiety linked to the past. As for the future-oriented anxiety, I'd like to quote my dad, who told me from the time I was a little girl that, "99% of what you worry about never happens anyway." And he's right. If you've ever rehearsed a difficult conversation in your head before actually talking to someone, then you know things rarely go as we plan. At least, not in the exact way we plan. Sure, that conversation will be hard, but it's not like the person actually said the things you rehearsed for them in your own head!

When you catch yourself dwelling on something you can't change (Why did I say that? Did I sound stupid?) or imagining worst-case scenarios (What if I fail? What if everything goes wrong?), remember that neither of these thought patterns serve you—they only drain more of your mental and emotional energy. This is why burnout and anxiety create a vicious cycle. When you're burned out, you don't have the emotional reserves to manage stress effectively. So, your brain kicks into high alert, trying to anticipate every possible disaster in an effort to regain control. But instead of solving the problem, it just keeps you stuck in a constant state of tension.

One way to break the cycle is to pause and breathe. Our controlled, even breath tells our bodies that we're safe and secure. It's one of the reasons I use the breath as a tool as often as possible. It's accessible, and it works. Breathe and think about what's currently happening. Is the thing you're worried about legit? If so, then how can you take action to make things better? Action is an antidote to anxiety, my friend, and it will help you move through it.

If you can't take action on what's troubling you, then what can you take action on? What in the current moment can help you feel more secure and in control? Sometimes it's helpful to journal out your thoughts, or if you're the praying type, spending some time in prayer can help.

Burnout thrives on chronic stress, and anxiety is one of the biggest stress amplifiers. By managing anxiety, you're not just easing your mind—you're also helping to prevent burnout from taking an even bigger toll on your well-being.

Resentment

If you hated group projects as much as I did, you know the feeling of resentment. It's almost inevitable, especially if you were the one who always stepped up to take charge of the assignment while others coasted.

Resentment is a beast of an emotion, yet like anger and anxiety, it holds important information. It builds when we feel wronged or taken advantage of, but don't address it. Maybe it's because we don't want to rock the boat. Maybe we convince ourselves it wasn't a big deal. Maybe we hope someone else will say something first. But the problem is, when resentment goes unspoken, it festers—and over time, it can lead straight to burnout.

Women, in particular, are conditioned to downplay our hurt feelings. We tell ourselves: *Maybe he didn't mean it that way. Maybe she'll realize on her own. Maybe I'm just overreacting.* The reality is, if someone pushes an unreasonable deadline, takes credit for your work, or disrespects you and you don't speak up, they're likely to do it again. Not because they're a bad person, but because most people are focused on their own needs.

Let's say your boss asks you to work late once. You agree, even though it frustrates you. The next time it happens, you feel a little more irritated. By the third time, you feel taken advantage of. By the fourth time, you're downright mad. If this cycle continues, resentment sets in—and burnout follows. What started as a manageable frustration morphs into bitterness and exhaustion. Suddenly, you're fantasizing about quitting, feeling drained by even the thought of work, and struggling to find any motivation.

Resentment is like anger with an added layer of bitterness. It doesn't just make you mad—it makes you feel stuck. It convinces you there's no way out except an explosion (hopefully not literally!). I get it. I've been there. And it sneaks up faster than you think.

The key is communication, with others and with yourself. Many resentment-inducing situations could be avoided with clearer boundaries and honest conversations. And that starts with recognizing what you will and won't tolerate. If something feels unfair, don't sweep it under the rug. Address it before resentment snowballs into burnout.

Frustration

Frustration often comes bundled with anger and a dash of helplessness. Just like the other emotions we've talked about though, frustration has something important to tell us. It highlights what's lacking or, to put a more empowering spin on it, it reveals when we want something more.

Maybe you're frustrated because you want more time for yourself, but your schedule is packed with obligations. Maybe you want more respect at work, but you're constantly being overlooked. Maybe you want more energy, but chronic exhaustion keeps dragging you down. Whatever it is, frustration is a signal that something isn't aligned.

As women, we overcommit out of habit. We say yes when we mean no because we don't want to upset anyone. People-pleasing feels safer especially when someone else's anger could be dangerous or unpredictable. Instead of setting clear boundaries, we say "maybe" to avoid conflict, dragging out decisions until we're stretched too thin. This cycle of self-sacrifice and avoidance can build into burnout-inducing frustration.

Frustration can also stem from our physical health. Many people are still dealing with the lingering effects of long Covid, myself included. I get so frustrated when I can't find the right word in conversation. It's something that never used to happen to me, and now, at times, it feels like my brain is stuck in second gear.

Here's the thing about frustration: it signals a blockage. Maybe it's a blocked path to something you want. Maybe it's a blocked connection between your energy levels and your obligations. Maybe, like me, it's a blocked neural pathway keeping you from finding the word you need. Whatever the case, frustration isn't just random irritation—it's information.

So, what's driving your frustration? If it's a communication issue with your partner, maybe it's time to schedule an appointment with a therapist. If you're frustrated by exhaustion, take a step back and look at your schedule. Are you overloading yourself? Pushing past your limits? Frustration is your body's way of waving a red flag so pay attention before it turns into something bigger.

Grief

One of the hardest human emotions is grief. Even the most introverted among us are social creatures. The great moments in life often include others, whether we're sharing them in real-time or simply telling the story later. Holidays, vacations, work anniversaries—all of these milestones carry a social aspect. So when we lose someone, or there's a major shift in our family structure, even the most ordinary routines, like a morning commute, feel different. Grief is more than just sadness. It's disorientation. It's an adjustment to a world that no longer looks or feels the same.

Grief is universal, yet in Western culture, we're often conditioned to suppress it. In some parts of the world, grieving out loud—keening, wailing, fully expressing the depth of loss—is considered both common and respectful. Here? We're expected to keep it together. We nod politely at funerals, offer a tight-lipped "sheesh" smile, and try to move on. Especially in the South, where repressing emotions is often mistaken for good manners.

I've always struggled at funerals. I leave with a pounding headache—not because of the loss itself, but because I don't feel like I can express my feelings. As an empath, I absorb the emotions around me, and the weight of all that unspoken grief feels oppressive.

But grief isn't just about death. It's also about change. We grieve the loss of a marriage, a friendship, or even a sense of identity. Parents grieve when their kids go off to college. Caregivers grieve while watching a loved one decline. Grief, the emotion, can hit like a ton of bricks. But grieving, the process, is what unfolds over time.

And here's where burnout comes in: Unprocessed grief is exhausting. When we don't allow ourselves to feel and move through it, we pile more stress onto an already overloaded system. We force ourselves to "get over it" for the comfort of others, all while silently carrying the weight. Remember, burnout thrives on unacknowledged emotions. If we don't take the time to grieve, it will manifest in other ways—fatigue, irritability, even physical illness.

Grief is both emotional and primal. Honoring it, instead of suppressing it, is an act of self-compassion. It doesn't mean wallowing, and it doesn't mean you'll feel this way forever. But giving yourself permission to grieve, without shame, without apology, prevents emotional buildup that could otherwise lead to burnout down the road.

So take care of you. You don't have to perform strength for anyone else's comfort.

Excitement

You know that feeling you get on the first day of a new job? The butterflies in your stomach, the thrill of a fresh start, the belief that *this* opportunity is going to be the best ever? Sometimes, it truly is. Excitement is a powerful, energizing force but it can also contribute to burnout.

When we dive into something new with enthusiasm, it's easy to get caught up in the whirlwind. We're super motivated, super driven, and super engaged. And any high-intensity emotion, whether positive or negative, can leave us feeling tapped out. We tend to focus on how anger, anxiety, and fear can exhaust us, but equally intense emotions like excitement, elation, and joy can drain us just as much.

Excitement and overstimulation also go hand-in-hand. Think about the last time you attended a wedding or a big party, something fun, social, and nonstop. By the end, you were probably exhausted. That's because the brain doesn't differentiate between emotional arousal and stress. The same amygdala activation that kicks in during fight-flight-freeze-or-fawn mode is also triggered by excitement. Just as your brain can't always tell the difference between the "danger signal" of a stressful email and an actual predator, it also doesn't distinguish between excitement-stress and distress. The nervous system just registers heightened arousal, and if we don't give ourselves time to recover, we burn out.

So while it's tempting to go all-in on a new job, project, or passion with boundless energy, it's important to pace yourself. Enjoy the excitement, but make sure you're not overextending your energy. Set boundaries around rest, allow yourself downtime, and remember that even positive stress is still stress.

Cynicism

I was the most cynical teenager. I mean, *John Hughes characters stuck in detention* levels of cynical. So, trust me, I know this emotion well. Cynicism is often one of the earliest warning signs of burnout.

You might notice yourself doubting that your coworkers will actually follow through on what they promised. You start believing that no one is really listening to you. You catch yourself thinking that people are just out for themselves, that companies don't care, that everything is rigged in favor of those at the top.

Cynicism isn't necessarily wrong. There are selfish people and exploitative companies out there. But when cynicism becomes your default perspective, it's a sign that you're heading toward burnout. It shifts from being a reasonable response to a specific situation to an all-encompassing filter that colors everything in negativity and distrust.

Here's where I want to reiterate: burnout is not your fault. It's often caused by systems, workplaces, and environments that are failing the people within them. And yes, in many cases, your workplace is to blame. A truly good leader takes responsibility for their team's well-being and does everything possible to prevent burnout. Unfortunately, not all leaders do.

So, if you're feeling cynical, don't ignore it. It's a signal that something needs to change. Maybe you need a new job. Maybe you need to set firmer boundaries at work. Maybe you need to unplug from the constant onslaught of political news. Whatever it is, listen to your cynicism but don't let it consume you. When it takes over completely, cynicism stops being useful and starts becoming its own kind of burnout.

Overwhelm

"Stressed is being in the weeds. Overwhelmed is being blown."[3]

You could say overwhelm lives somewhere between stress and full burnout—it's that sense of being completely buried, as if everything is moving faster and faster while you're stuck in slow motion, unable to keep up.

Overwhelm doesn't just show up when your to-do list is too long. It can come from emotions, thoughts, anxiety, external expectations, or even the weight of the world's problems (and let's be real—the world has *a lot* of problems these days). It's

---

3. Brown, *Atlas of the Heart*, 8.

that crushing feeling that no matter how much you do, it won't be enough.

Overwhelm can creep up suddenly or build over time, and if it isn't addressed, it can snowball into full burnout. It leads to brain fog, anxiety, and decision paralysis—as if your brain just shuts down under the pressure. And yet, the way out of overwhelm is often the very thing that feels the least natural: slowing down.

That's the cruel trick of overwhelm. Our nervous system tells us to go faster, to push harder, to *fix it all right now*. But that only makes things worse. Think of overwhelm like quicksand—the more you struggle against it, the deeper you sink. The way out isn't frantic effort; it's stillness, breath, and small, intentional steps forward.

Fear

Like shame, fear is a universal experience, not just because we're taught to be afraid, but because fear is hardwired into our neurobiology. The fight-flight-freeze-or-fawn response is present at birth. Have you ever seen a startled baby? They freeze, contract their little bodies, then cry in an automatic survival response. Our brains are constantly scanning for threats, looking for errors in the environment. That hyper-awareness helped our ancestors avoid predators and dangers, but in today's world, it can keep us in a perpetual state of stress, even when there's no immediate threat.

And here's the thing: burnout and fear are deeply intertwined.

As we edge closer to burnout, fear is often the force that keeps us pushing forward, even when our bodies and souls are begging for relief. Fear of losing our home, our job, our security. Fear of letting people down. Fear of losing status, autonomy, or purpose. These fears whisper that if we slow down, we'll fall behind. If we stop, we'll lose everything. So we keep running on empty, ignoring the warning signs until we crash.

Fear is rapid-fire; it happens before we even realize it's there. That's why the antidote to fear is the same as the antidote to overwhelm: slow down. Pause and assess the situation. Instead of spiraling into anxiety about the past or the future, assess your current situation. What are you actually afraid of right now? Is there a real, immediate danger—or just the fear of what might happen? If your fear could speak, what would it tell you? What does it want you to know?

Fear is an instinct, but it doesn't have to be in the driver's seat. When we learn to recognize it, not as an enemy, but as a messenger, we can start making choices from wisdom instead of panic.

Hopelessness

Hope is a driving force in our lives. It keeps us going, pushing us to persevere, believe in goodness, and trust that things can get better. As Brené Brown writes, *"We need hope like we need air."*[4] And when hope is gone? Hopelessness sucks the air right out of your body.

---

4. Ibid, 97.

That's why hopelessness is such a devastating emotional state. When you're burned out, hope can feel impossible to access. You've tried everything, and nothing seems to change. You can't catch a break. The stress, exhaustion, and pressure feel endless.

Interestingly, Brown argues that hope isn't an emotion, it's a learned skill.[5] We build hope through struggle but when that struggle feels insurmountable, hopelessness sets in. And when burnout fuels that hopelessness, it's easy to believe that no amount of effort will make a difference. That your goals are out of reach. That your relationships are broken beyond repair. That nothing will ever change.

But here's the truth: no one is without help. No situation is completely unchangeable. Hopelessness may feel final, but it's a sign that something needs to shift. Maybe it's your circumstances. Maybe it's your mindset. Maybe it's the support systems around you. But hope isn't lost, it just needs space to breathe again.

Guilt

Guilt and shame often go hand in hand, but they aren't the same. Shame whispers, "You're a bad person." Guilt says, "You did something bad." Or, in the case of many women, guilt says you didn't do what you "should" have done.

Anyone who has experienced "mom guilt" knows this feeling all too well. Mothers feel guilty for what they've done, what

---

5. Ibid, 101.

they haven't done, and what they believe they *should* have done. But it's not just moms—this cycle of guilt is ingrained in so many of us. We feel guilty for taking time for ourselves, for setting boundaries, for saying no.

Burnout and guilt are deeply intertwined. The more burned out we become, the more guilt creeps in. We feel guilty for not working harder, for not being more available, for not meeting unrealistic expectations. And when guilt lingers too long, it often morphs into shame—into the belief that we're failing, that we're not enough.

Like all the emotions we've covered before it, guilt is a signal, not a sentence. It can serve as a guide, nudging us toward necessary changes. But it should never be used as proof that you're failing or unworthy. If guilt is weighing you down, ask yourself: Is this guilt rooted in truth, or is it tied to impossible expectations? Because, my friend, you are not bad. You are not failing. You deserve the same grace you give to others.

Bringing It All Together

If we're going to break up with burnout, we need to shine a light on the unexamined forces that push us to keep going, even when we're running on empty. The emotions tied to burnout—anger, anxiety, guilt, frustration, cynicism, and more—aren't just random reactions. They are signals, telling us where we're overextended, where our boundaries are too loose, and where we need change.

When we don't recognize these emotions for what they are, we get stuck. Frustration turns into resentment. Guilt turns into overwork. Anxiety turns into perfectionism. And before we know it, we're caught in a cycle of burnout without fully understanding why. But when we shift our perspective—when we stop seeing these emotions as burdens and start recognizing them as guideposts—we take back our power.

So, what now?

First, hold yourself in compassion. You're human, and these emotions are part of the deal. Nothing you're feeling is wrong, it's all just information.

Second, get curious. Instead of judging yourself for feeling overwhelmed, anxious, or resentful, ask: *Why? What is this emotion trying to tell me?*

And finally, look deeper. The problem often isn't the problem. If you're snapping at loved ones, is it really about them, or are you exhausted? If you're feeling cynical at work, is it because you don't care—or because you've been carrying too much for too long?

Burnout is a direct result of disconnection—from yourself, your values, your joy. By recognizing your emotions as guideposts instead of burdens, you can begin to break free.

Now that we've unpacked how burnout manifests and what it feels like, it's time to look at the bigger picture: your burnout patterns. In the next chapter, we'll explore how different types of burnout overlap, reinforce each other, and create unique burnout cycles. Because once you understand how burnout plays out for *you*, you can finally start making real, lasting changes.

13

Identify Your Burnout Pattern

B y now, you've explored the six types of burnout and the emotions that fuel them. And if you're like most people, you probably saw yourself in more than one. That's because burnout doesn't happen in isolation—it's a pattern, a tangled web of experiences and emotions that shape how we respond to stress.

For some, burnout starts in one area and cascades into others. Maybe it begins as mental burnout, but the overwhelm spirals into emotional exhaustion and eventually physical burnout. Or perhaps empathic burnout drains you so much that even social interactions feel unbearable. No matter where it begins, burnout doesn't exist in neat little categories —it intertwines, deepens, and shifts based on your experiences, emotions, stressors, and personal tendencies.

The goal of this chapter isn't just to help you recognize burnout—it's to help you recognize *your* burnout. While I've outlined the emotions that often trigger or signal each type of burnout, this isn't a rigid framework; it's a guide. Burnout is deeply personal, and only you can determine what resonates most with your experience.

So before we dive in, take a moment to reflect:

- Which burnout types resonated most with you?
- Do you notice a pattern in how burnout manifests in your life?
- Which emotions—anger, anxiety, frustration, guilt, cynicism, or overwhelm—seem to fuel your burnout cycle?

If you're unsure, don't worry. As we go through each type again—this time integrating the emotional layers and connections between burnout types—you'll start to see your patterns more clearly. And once you do, you'll have the awareness you need to start breaking the cycle before it takes hold.

Social Burnout: When People Feel Like Too Much

Social burnout happens when you've just hit your limit with people. Even interactions you'd normally enjoy feel exhausting. Social situations become overwhelming, and you just want to curl up under a weighted blanket and hide from the world.

Social burnout isn't just about needing alone time. It's about feeling drained by the presence or expectations of others— whether in person, online, or even in your own home.

The Emotional Landscape of Social Burnout

Trigger Emotions (What Fuels Social Burnout?)

- Obligation – Feeling pressured to show up, even when you don't want to.
- Guilt – Worrying that saying no makes you a bad friend, parent, partner, or coworker.
- Anxiety – Anticipating social exhaustion before it even happens.

Burnout Signals (What Tells You Social Burnout Has Set In?)

- Irritation – Small things that wouldn't normally bother you now feel unbearable.
- Resentment – Feeling like people expect too much from you.
- Apathy – Social events and relationships you usually enjoy feel like an energy drain.

How Social Burnout Connects to Other Burnout Types

- Emotional Burnout – When you're socially drained, your patience, empathy, and resilience take a hit, leading to frustration, guilt, or resentment toward others.
- Energetic Burnout – If you're sensitive to emotions (hello, empaths), even being around people can feel

like an energy drain—even when you're not actively engaging.

- Mental Burnout – The constant processing of social cues, small talk, and obligations can leave your brain feeling fried, making even simple decisions feel exhausting.

Is Social Burnout Part of Your Burnout Pattern?

Remember, introverts and extroverts both experience social burnout. Look back at past times when you've felt overwhelmed, anxious, or completely drained.

- Were you juggling too many social obligations?
- Did the pressure to be "on" contribute to your stress?
- Did you keep saying yes to things you didn't actually want to do?
- When you finally got alone time, did you feel guilty for needing it?

Mental Burnout: When Your Brain Is Full

Mental burnout happens when you've absorbed too much information and processed too many decisions. Your brain feels overloaded—like a computer with too many tabs open, running too many programs at once. You're mentally exhausted, and even simple tasks feel overwhelming.

But mental burnout isn't just about too much information—it's about not having enough space to process it. Whether it's work demands, endless decision-making, or social media overload, your brain never gets a break.

The Emotional Landscape of Mental Burnout

Trigger Emotions (What Fuels Mental Burnout?)

- Overwhelm – Feeling mentally flooded, like there's too much coming at you at once.
- Anxiety – The pressure to keep up, stay informed, and make the "right" decisions.
- Fear – Worrying about making mistakes or failing to meet expectations.

Burnout Signals (What Tells You Mental Burnout Has Set In?)

- Frustration – Feeling short-tempered, like everything is just "too much."
- Anger – Reacting more sharply than usual, snapping at interruptions or minor mistakes.
- Cynicism – Losing faith in your work, feeling like nothing you do really matters.

How Mental Burnout Connects to Other Burnout Types

- Emotional Burnout – When your brain is overloaded, emotional regulation suffers. Instead of processing feelings, you might shut down or feel emotionally detached.

- Physical Burnout – Mental fatigue disrupts sleep, and lack of sleep makes mental burnout worse, creating a vicious cycle.
- Social Burnout – Social interactions require mental processing—if your brain is maxed out, even casual conversations feel exhausting.

Is Mental Burnout Part of Your Burnout Pattern?

Think about the last time you felt completely mentally drained:

- Were you constantly making decisions, juggling responsibilities, or absorbing too much information?
- Did overthinking leave you feeling exhausted before you even took action?
- Did you struggle to turn off your brain, even when you wanted to rest?
- Did frustration, anger, or cynicism take over, making you snap at others or withdraw?

Physical Burnout: When Your Body Taps Out

Physical burnout happens when your body is exhausted—whether from too little rest, too much stress, or pushing yourself beyond your limits. Your body is running on fumes, and no amount of caffeine or "powering through" can fix it.

Unlike regular fatigue, physical burnout doesn't just go away with a good night's sleep. It's your body waving red flags and demanding real recovery. If ignored, it can escalate into chronic fatigue, injury, or illness.

The Emotional Landscape of Physical Burnout

Trigger Emotions (What Fuels Physical Burnout?)

- Excitement – Overextending yourself because you're passionate about something.
- Obligation – Feeling like you have to keep going, even when your body begs for rest.
- Fear – Worrying that slowing down means falling behind, losing momentum, or being seen as weak.

Burnout Signals (What Tells You Physical Burnout Has Set In?)

- Frustration – Feeling like your body is betraying you when exhaustion takes over.
- Resentment – Pushing through pain or fatigue and blaming yourself (or others) for your condition.
- Irritability – Small inconveniences feel unbearable because your body is depleted.

How Physical Burnout Connects to Other Burnout Types

- Emotional Burnout – When your body is exhausted, your ability to regulate emotions suffers.

Small stressors feel bigger, and you may feel emotionally reactive or completely numb.

- Mental Burnout – Exhaustion makes it harder to think clearly, remember things, or stay focused. Your brain struggles just as much as your body.
- Energetic Burnout – Physical depletion can lead to an overall sense of misalignment, making you feel disconnected from yourself and your environment.

Is Physical Burnout Part of Your Burnout Pattern?

Think about how you handle rest and recovery:

- Do you ignore exhaustion until you crash?
- Do you feel guilty for resting—even when you're drained?
- When you're physically burned out, do you notice mood swings, irritability, or emotional numbness?

Emotional Burnout: When You Can't Feel Anymore

Emotional burnout tends to creep in after prolonged emotional labor—whether from caregiving, navigating a difficult relationship, or simply dealing with the highs and lows of life. It often follows major life changes, intense social obligations (think: holidays or family events), or an extended period of stress where you've had to hold it together for others.

Emotional burnout happens when you've been carrying too much for too long. It's not just about feeling overwhelmed—it's about feeling nothing at all. You might start out emotionally drained, but over time, that exhaustion turns into numbness. Things that used to move you—joy, sadness, excitement—now feel distant, like you're watching life happen instead of experiencing it.

But emotional burnout isn't just about detachment. It's about the weight of emotions—yours and everyone else's—becoming too heavy to hold. If you're the person who's always there for others, always supporting, always holding things together, you might find yourself here.

The Emotional Landscape of Emotional Burnout

Trigger Emotions (What Fuels Emotional Burnout?)

- Grief – The exhaustion that follows prolonged sadness or loss, even if that loss isn't tangible.
- Obligation – Feeling like you *have* to keep showing up emotionally, even when you have nothing left to give.
- Helplessness – A growing sense that no matter what you do, things won't change.

Burnout Signals (What Tells You Emotional Burnout Has Set In?)

- Apathy – You don't feel as much, and you don't care that you don't care.
- Cynicism – You expect the worst and assume things won't get better.
- Anger – Small frustrations escalate quickly because your emotional reserves are depleted.

How Emotional Burnout Connects to Other Burnout Types

- Empathic Burnout – Constantly taking on others' pain can push you toward emotional shutdown, making it hard to connect or care.
- Social Burnout – Emotional burnout often leads to withdrawal from social interactions because engaging feels exhausting.
- Physical Burnout – Carrying heavy emotions takes a toll on your body. Unprocessed emotional stress can show up as headaches, digestive issues, fatigue, and chronic tension.

Is Emotional Burnout Part of Your Burnout Pattern?

- Do you feel emotionally numb—like you're just going through the motions?
- Are you the person others turn to for support, while you rarely get to be the one receiving care?

- Have you been through a string of emotionally demanding life events with no time to recover?
- Do you work in a highly emotional profession (healthcare, social work, public service)?
- Do you feel like you have to push your emotions down to keep functioning?

Energetic Burnout: When Everything Feels Too Heavy

Energetic burnout happens when you've been absorbing too much—whether from an event, other people's emotions, or deep personal transformation. Unlike emotional burnout, which stems from personal stressors, energetic burnout is about external absorption. If you've ever felt like you're carrying the weight of others, or like your energy is completely drained after a big experience, this type of burnout may resonate with you.

The Emotional Landscape of Energetic Burnout

Trigger Emotions (What Fuels Energetic Burnout?)

- Overwhelm – Too much external energy, input, or expectation at once.
- Guilt – Feeling like you *should* hold space for others, even when you're drained.
- Resentment – The frustration of giving too much and having nothing left for yourself.

Burnout Signals (What Tells You Energetic Burnout Has Set In?)

- Apathy – Emotional dullness, like you're disconnected from your own needs.
- Exhaustion – You feel drained, but it's not just physical—it's a full-body depletion.
- Irritability – Even minor interactions feel intrusive or overstimulating.

How Energetic Burnout Connects to Other Burnout Types

- Social Burnout – Large gatherings, retreats, or back-to-back events can drain your energy reserves, making even enjoyable interactions feel depleting.
- Empathic Burnout – If you absorb emotions from others, your energy field can become overloaded, leading to disconnection and exhaustion.
- Mental Burnout – A cluttered energetic space often mirrors a cluttered mind. If your energy is scattered, focusing and processing information can feel impossible.

Is Energetic Burnout Part of Your Burnout Pattern?

- Do you feel completely wiped out after social events—even ones you looked forward to?
- Have you ever attended a retreat, conference, or large gathering and needed days to recover?

- Do you struggle to tell the difference between your own emotions and the energy you've absorbed from others?
- Are you in a profession or role where you hold space for others (coaching, therapy, energy work, leadership)?
- Do you feel like your energy is scattered, ungrounded, or detached from yourself?

Empathic Burnout: When You Just Can't Care Anymore

Empathic burnout happens when your capacity to care for others feels completely drained. Unlike emotional burnout, which stems from managing your own emotions, empathic burnout is about carrying the emotions of others—often to the point of depletion. You might feel disconnected from people's struggles, overwhelmed by the weight of suffering in the world, or simply unable to summon the energy to care in the way you once did.

The Emotional Landscape of Empathic Burnout

Trigger Emotions (What Fuels Empathic Burnout?)

- Sadness – Being constantly exposed to suffering can take a deep emotional toll.
- Helplessness – Feeling powerless to help or fix the pain you see around you.

- Overwhelm – Carrying too much emotional weight —yours and everyone else's.

Burnout Signals (What Tells You Empathic Burnout Has Set In?)

- Apathy – You don't have the energy to care, and you're too exhausted to feel guilty about it.
- Irritation – You become easily frustrated by other people's problems or emotions.
- Cynicism – You start feeling like nothing really matters, or that people's struggles are futile.

How Empathic Burnout Connects to Other Burnout Types

- Emotional Burnout – The constant absorption of others' struggles can leave you emotionally depleted, making it hard to process your own emotions.
- Energetic Burnout – Taking on too much emotional energy from others can leave you feeling ungrounded, disconnected, and exhausted in a way that rest doesn't fix.
- Social Burnout – If being around people means constantly managing their emotions, social interactions can become overwhelming, leading to avoidance or withdrawal.

Is Empathic Burnout Part of Your Burnout Pattern?

- Do you find yourself emotionally shutting down when confronted with others' struggles?
- Do you work in a caregiving or service role (healthcare, therapy, social work, teaching)?
- Have you ever felt guilty for not caring as much as you used to?
- Does watching the news or hearing about injustice make you feel hopeless instead of motivated?
- Do you feel emotionally drained from constantly supporting friends or family?

The Path to Breaking Free

Burnout isn't a single event—it's a cycle. And like any cycle, it has a pattern, a rhythm, and a set of predictable triggers. Now that you've explored the different types of burnout, the emotions that fuel them, and the ways they overlap, you're in a position of power. You can start recognizing the early warning signs. You can spot where burnout sneaks up on you. You can understand what drains you the fastest and where you need to set firmer boundaries.

But awareness alone isn't enough. Knowing your burnout pattern is just the first step—breaking the pattern is where the real work begins.

In the next section, we'll move beyond recognizing burnout and into breaking up with burnout for good. We'll explore how to shift your mindset, reclaim your energy, and set boundaries that actually work. Because burnout doesn't have to be your normal. And you, my friend, are not here just to survive—you're here to thrive.

PART III

Breaking Up With Burnout

14

Mindset Shifts for Burnout Recovery

B reaking up with burnout isn't just about adding self-care routines or setting better boundaries, although we'll definitely talk about those—it's about shifting the way you think. Many of us have internalized beliefs that keep us stuck in cycles of overwork, emotional exhaustion, and self-doubt. These beliefs tell us that we have to be perfect, that we have to push through discomfort, or that we have to control everything around us to be successful. So before we dive into strategies for breaking the cycle, we need to get a few things straight.

These reminders will help you reframe your mindset, let go of the thought patterns that keep you trapped, and open yourself up to a more sustainable way of living. Some of these will feel simple, but simple isn't always easy. Consider them your foundation as you begin the real work of breaking up with burnout.

Drop the Expectations

One of the tenets of Buddhism that has always struck me is the idea that expectations cause suffering. Think about it—how many times have you entered a situation with specific expectations, only to be disappointed? How did that feel?

A key to breaking up with burnout is learning to shift your expectations. Take a moment to reflect: What are your expectations for your tasks, your job, your relationships—hell, even your day-to-day life? Now, consider loosening your grip on them. I know what you're thinking: *"Wait a minute, Megan! Are you saying I should lower my expectations?"* Nope. I'm saying you should aim to release them altogether. Boundaries? Yes, absolutely. But rigid expectations? Those can fast-track you to emotional burnout.

Let me give you an example. Imagine you're heading into a meeting—maybe it's a PTA meeting, a boardroom discussion, or a team check-in. It doesn't really matter which; what matters is your attitude and expectations. You have three choices:

1. You can go into it expecting conflict, mentally bracing for someone to whine about a problem or push back. You're stressed before it even begins.
2. You can go into it expecting to sway everyone to your opinion, be the darling of the meeting, and leave ready to share margaritas with your favorite PTA mom/coworker/friend/whatever.

3. You go in neutral, without expectations of good or bad—just open, curious, and engaged in the moment.

Which option do you think is the healthiest? Which one is the hardest? Spoiler alert: the answer to both is option three.

I get it—it's tempting to lean into drama, whether it's preparing for a fight or indulging in an unrealistic fantasy of how things *should* go. The brain craves novelty and wants to be entertained pretty much all the time. What's more entertaining than a fight at the elementary school over a pizza fundraiser? Drama is why the Kardashians exist.

Finding the neutrality in a situation takes practice. The next time you find yourself revving up for conflict or having cotton candy and unicorn dreams about something going your way, take a pause. Breathe. Get back into your body. Remind yourself that things may not unfold as you expect— and that's okay. That's the key: *It's okay for things to go differently than you imagined.*

Perhaps most importantly—if something doesn't go as planned, it's not a reflection of your worth as a human being. You are not your outcomes.

Emotions Just Are

Emotions just are. Feelings just are. You are not a bad person for experiencing a so-called "negative" emotion.

Remember, the patriarchy and systems of white supremacy have long dictated how we should behave—what's "acceptable" and what's not. And for too many of us, "acceptable" means keeping quiet and looking pretty. Screw that.

Anger is holy. Fear is sacred. Disdain has something to tell you. Emotions are an essential part of the human experience —and they have nothing to do with your worth.

Instead of trying to rationalize your emotions, try feeling them. Observe them. Make note of them. And—most importantly—pay attention to what caused them. Your emotions are messengers, and when you stop dismissing them, you'll uncover an understanding of yourself that's unlike anything else.

Perfectionism is Toxic

Perfectionism is a poison, and here's the reality: there is no such thing as perfect. Most of the time, we don't even realize we're falling into the perfectionism trap. We perceive perfection through comparison—measuring ourselves against others and deciding that they're doing it "right" while we're falling short.

I'll never forget the first time I heard, "Don't compare yourself to people on the internet. They're only posting the highlight reel." It hit me like a ton of bricks. Of course, it's true! Yet we still get sucked into the illusion. Stop worrying about how things look and start focusing on how they feel. Keep your eyes on your own paper.

That said, it's important to notice when the little perfectionism voice pops up. What is it saying? Where does it come from? What messages—internal or external—are feeding it? What childhood stories are creeping into your present reality?

Perfectionism isn't about being flawless—it's about fear. Fear of not being good enough. Fear of judgment. Fear of disappointing others. Instead of chasing the impossible, get curious: What's behind your urge to be perfect? Because once you understand that, you can finally start letting it go.

What's In Your Control?

Burnout thrives in the space between what we want to control and what we actually can control. The more energy we spend trying to manage the unmanageable, the more drained we become. That's why one of the most important things you can do in breaking up with burnout is to get clear on where your energy is going—and whether it's being wasted on things beyond your influence.

So, what is in your control? You have a say in how you structure your schedule (to some extent), what you eat, what you listen to, and how you spend your time. You can control how you respond to situations, even if you can't always control what happens. On the flip side, there's plenty you can't control, like the weather, traffic, or the latest Mercury-in-retrograde drama. You also can't control other people's choices, how they perceive you, or whether they decide to like you.

Yes, we should all strive to be *not* an asshole. But even in our best moments, someone, somewhere, will decide they don't like us. And guess what? That's okay. Burnout often comes from fighting battles that aren't ours to fight, pouring energy into things that won't change just because we want them to. So, where in your life are you trying to control the uncontrollable? Where are you spending energy that could be better used elsewhere?

15

Your Brain is Basically Playdough

I remember the first time I met my younger self. It was during a meditation session for an emerging modality that a friend of mine was teaching. The modality, called Neurosculpting®, combines traditional meditation practices with neuroscience to rewrite the scripts in the mind. Wrapped in one of my many shawls, sitting on a meditation cushion in a hand-built ashram studio (literally built by its owner, with his own two hands), I met younger me.

Her name is Meggie—the nickname my dad used a handful of times throughout my childhood, but it stuck with me as the identifier for this little, scared part of myself.

What was she scared of? Being left all alone. I began to cry silently right there on the meditation cushion. This was before I'd learned any of the tools and modalities I practice today, but instinctively, I wrapped her in my arms and told her that I would never leave her. She was safe with me. And it was on that day that a small part of my long-held fears melted away.

I share this story to demonstrate that yes, while we're conditioned to act and be a certain way, that conditioning can be rewritten.

Rather than holding onto old ideas about who we "have" to be, what if we actually met ourselves? What if we developed a relationship with the little parts of our personality that carry our past fears and insecurities? Yes, I'm telling you to literally talk to yourself. No, you're not crazy.

In the 1970s, Dr. Richard Schwartz noticed a pattern in the way people spoke about their emotions. He was studying family systems therapy when he realized that people naturally refer to different aspects of themselves in conversation. He's a family therapist and academic, so he went about developing this new approach—Internal Family Systems (IFS)—systematically and scientifically, which I really appreciate. If you've ever said something like, "A part of me is glad our trip got rescheduled," then you've already touched on the foundation of his work.

Schwartz developed IFS based on this exact way of speaking, recognizing that our personalities are made up of different "parts"—many of which hold old wounds from childhood. This concept isn't new, but Schwartz's contribution was in recognizing that each part of us has its own fears, concerns, and emotional scars. And, more importantly, that these parts can heal.

You don't have to dive deep into IFS to practice it. In fact, you've already started. When we spoke to shame, we acknowledged it as a separate part of ourselves—one that carries pain, but isn't the whole of who we are. Now, let's take it a step further.

The key is developing a relationship with our parts, and it's easier than you think. When you find yourself thinking a thought like, "I'm not good enough," or "I should..."—pause. Before trying to rationalize it away, see if you can feel where it lives in your body. Our bodies are like radars for internal information—they register emotions before our brains even process them. I bet if you and I were sitting across from each other, and I asked, "Where do you carry stress in your body?" you'd be able to tell me right off.

I carry mental stress between my shoulders and my upper back while energetic stress clusters in the bottoms of my feet, which I'm sure a reflexologist could shed some light on. When either of these areas ache, I know there's something stressing me out, even if my brain isn't sure what it is! Your stress has a physical home too.

When you identify where this stress is hanging out in your body, try asking it: "What do you want me to know?" And then, here's the magic, you actually have to listen.

We'll explore this more in later chapters, but here's what I want you to take away for now:

Getting through the stress and the pressures of patriarchy, toxic capitalism—hell, even voting season—is a lot easier when you listen to your body. When it's tired, listen. When there are butterflies in your stomach, pause and ask yourself: Am I excited? Nervous? Anxious?

It might sound a little out there at first, but I promise, as you build this connection, your body will start communicating with you more and more. And the more your body communicates, the more you know what is true for you. This is how you begin to dismantle conditioning. So for now, your homework is simple: start talking to yourself.

Just maybe not out loud in crowded places...

16

Make Peace with Anxiety

M aking peace with anxiety is a process—one that isn't always easy, and sometimes, one we can't tackle alone. That's why I want to acknowledge this upfront: I take medication for my anxiety. I practice these tools, but I still experience anxiety on the regular. The goal isn't to eliminate it entirely. The goal is to manage it in a way that doesn't fuel burnout. Progress, not perfection.

Burnout and anxiety often go hand in hand. We discussed this relationship in more detail in the chapter on the emotions of burnout. As a reminder, anxiety can push us deeper into burnout by keeping us stuck in overthinking, second-guessing, and people-pleasing. It drains our mental energy, makes us hyper-aware of mistakes (both real and imagined), and keeps us in a state of emotional exhaustion.

The Time Stamp Exercise is one way to shift that pattern. It helps your brain recognize when a moment is over, so it stops replaying it on a loop.

The Time Stamp Exercise

The next time a memory from your past starts swirling in your mind—whether it's a cringe moment, an embarrassing misstep, or something you regret—pause and take a few deep breaths.

1. **Breathe in through your nose and out through your mouth.** Let the breath fill your belly and slow your nervous system down.
2. **Imagine the event written out on a large scroll.** You don't have to read it; just know that every detail is written there. (Mine always floats among the stars, but you can picture whatever feels right for you.)
3. **Look to the bottom of the scroll where there's a blank space.** On that line, imagine writing the day's date on it. If the event happened 10 years ago or you don't remember the exact details, that's fine. The goal is simply to date it. You can even use today's date.
4. **Stamp it.** Picture a giant, official stamp pressing into the scroll with a satisfying thud—something solid and final. The more detail you put into it, the more your brain registers it as complete.
5. **Send it off.** Imagine rolling up the scroll and sending it out into the universe. Maybe it gets burned up in the sun, torn to shreds, or dissolves into dust. Whatever makes it feel *gone* to you.

6. **Tell yourself:** *As of today, this no longer exists.* It's finished.

7. **Take a few more breaths and shake out your body.** Release the excess energy, physically signaling to your brain that you've let it go.

This takes practice, but over time, you'll find yourself unrolling a scroll anytime you need to let go of an old moment. It's been a game-changer for me—especially for those little things that pop up unexpectedly, like something awkward I said in a meeting or a moment I misunderstood.

And if all else fails? Remind yourself that most people are too focused on their own lives to remember your missteps. We're all wrapped up in our own worlds. That thing you're obsessing over? It's probably long forgotten by everyone else —if they even noticed it in the first place.

Burnout thrives on unprocessed emotions, and anxiety is one of its most relentless fuel sources. It keeps us in fight-or-flight mode, convinced we have to stay on high alert, overanalyze every decision, and anticipate every possible mistake. But the truth is, we can't recover from burnout if we're constantly bracing for impact.

Letting go of anxious loops and past regrets doesn't mean we stop caring—it means we free up energy for the things that actually matter. When we stop giving power to what's already over, we take a step closer to reclaiming our energy, our peace, and our sense of self. And that, my friend, is exactly how we start breaking up with burnout for good.

17

Align Your Life with What Really Matters

B urnout often stems from misalignment—when our time, energy, and obligations are spent in ways that don't reflect what truly matters to us. Without clarity on our values, we say yes to things that drain us, we push through exhaustion for external validation, and we let perfectionism override what actually fulfills us. Understanding your values helps you make decisions that protect your energy and reduce burnout before it starts.

Our values shape how we move through the world, often in ways we don't even realize. The gut reactions we have to certain situations, whether it's an instant sense of admiration or deep frustration, are fueled by our values. When we see something we love, or something that enrages us to the point of wanting to eliminate it from the world, our values are at play. Yet, for most of us, these guiding principles operate beneath the surface. They were instilled in us at a young age, and we rarely pause to consciously reflect on what they are or how they influence our choices.

In some ways, this automatic function is useful. We develop a sense of right and wrong, follow basic societal norms, and instinctively adhere to rules that keep us safe—like stopping at red lights and not going around kicking puppies. But when we move through life entirely on autopilot, we miss the opportunity to ensure that the way we spend our time and energy actually aligns with what matters most to us.

Your Values Support Your Energy Levels

Our values form the foundation of a life strategy for more happiness and satisfaction. When we make decisions aligned with our values, we reduce the stress of second-guessing ourselves. We stop wasting energy on things that don't serve us. Values create a built-in filter for protecting our energy from burnout-inducing commitments.

Think of making decisions like a decision tree, like the game "20 Questions." It's a process of asking yes/no questions to get to the answer. But what if you approached all decisions this way, intentionally consulting your values along the way? I originally designed this process for my business owner clients, only to realize it's just as relevant to our personal lives.

What if you made all your decisions like this?

Take the value "Trust Your Intuition." If you go into a job interview, you start with this value in mind. Let's say the interviewer mentions something about the office culture, which clashes with the remote work they advertised. Your intuition goes off. Do you ignore it, or do you ask questions about it?

Let's walk through that decision:

- You go into the interview conscious of your value: "Trust Your Intuition."
- The job posting said it was remote.
- The interviewer starts talking about office culture.
- That nagging gut feeling tells you something's not quite right.

Now, you have two choices:

1. Ignore your intuition and power through.
2. Honor your intuition, ask more questions about the office situation, and get clarity.

The harder choice is often the right one, the one that stays true to your values. The more you practice this, the easier it becomes.

When we understand our values and we've taken time to really recognize them, we're training our brains to pay more attention to little things in everyday life. The brain is a beautiful, pliable organ that can be molded according to our preferences. By paying attention to your values, you're actually training your brain to think in terms of these values. The new neural pathways that you create will become stronger the more you use them. In fact, they'll become so strong that it becomes easier to travel down those thought paths over time, and easier to think in terms of your values. If this sounds a lot like a mindfulness technique, 10 points! You're absolutely right.

What Are Your Values?

Are you scratching your head right now? Good. You're thinking. And yes, it can be daunting to answer such a hefty question as, "What are your values?" Let's break it down and simplify the process. Don't focus on your work or business values just yet. Start by thinking about your personal values. What are your guiding principles in life?

To give you an example, one of my guiding principles is: *You do what you say you're going to do.* To me, this means that I follow through on my commitments—whether it's picking up my partner's dry cleaning when I said I would or hitting a work deadline. I don't expect perfection of myself, just commitment and effort.

Now, take a moment to reflect on any guiding principles you hold. What are your non-negotiables? If nothing comes to mind, think about what irritates you. Often, we are irritated by others who fail to live up to one of our values. For instance, people who place high importance on honesty tend to have strong reactions when they are lied to.

Still unsure about where to start? Start by paying attention. When you make a decision, or something annoys you, make a note of it. It can be a mental note, or you can actually open your phone up and document it in your favorite notes app.

Be curious and non-judgmental about the decisions or your pet peeves. Why are you making that decision? Why does that behavior in someone else irritate you? You get the idea. Do this for a week and then sit down and think through the experience. This really is best done with a reflective tool like your journal. You can also use a dictation app to create some voice notes for yourself! Get creative with it.

When you review your experience, learn what you can from it. Think about the decisions you made for yourself and think about the ones that you made because you felt like you *should* make them. Any time the word "should" comes up, that's a sign that the value really isn't your own.

Another way to discern your values is to think about the times when you feel most proud of yourself. Yes, it's a good thing to be proud of yourself. It's the patriarchy that tells us we shouldn't be proud of ourselves. Think back over your past. When did you feel like you were really in the right? When did you feel proud of yourself for taking the difficult, but better, path? Those proud moments are clues about what's important to you...what you value.

This is a journey in both self-exploration and self-trust. Other people don't get to tell you what your values are. They don't get to tell you what's important. This is all you, babe. Here's a list of some values to help you think about them. Feel free to circle them, cross them out, make up your own... whatever works!

Adventurous	Dependable	Nimble
Agile	Driven	Open-minded
Aligned	Educated	Original
Altruistic	Empowered	Passionate
Ambitious	Energized	Patient
Analytical	Fair	Persistent
Approachable	Fearless	Proud
Artful	Forever-curious	Quirky
Balanced	Free	Relentless
Bold	Friendly	Resourceful
Brilliant	Generous	Respectful
Caring	Good-natured	Skilled
Collaborative	Gritty	Spontaneous
Committed	Honest	Surprising
Compassionate	Humble	Talented
Courageous	Inclusive	Tenacious
Courteous	Insightful	Unabashed
Credible	Intuitive	Weird
Curious	Invested	Without compromise
Delightful	Mindful	Zany

Create a list of your personal values, turn them in to guiding principles if that helps you activate them, then, grab a different color pen and circle the ones that also apply to your work or business. See what overlaps.

Why Are They Important to You?

Here's the last part of this exercise. As you consider your values, ask yourself why they're important to you. What does it mean to you if you adhere to each value? What emotions come up when you fulfill this value?

Burnout often happens when we try to control the uncontrollable—like other people's expectations or the relentless demands of hustle culture. Instead, focus on what is in your control: honoring your values, setting realistic expectations, and prioritizing where your energy goes based on what actually matters to you.

18

Boundaries are Your Friend

In today's world, we're dragged in so many different directions that we often feel like Elastigirl who's lost her stretch. We're just stretched out. Limp. Dragging our ass to the next thing on the list. There's this idea that others need us so much. And when we're in times of great societal stress, more people "need" things from us "right now." Honestly, I'm getting tired just thinking about it. But there are two things you can do that make all the difference in the world: modifying your schedule to serve your energy levels and setting—and keeping!—boundaries.

I'm going to shelve the former topic for Chapter 20 and focus on the latter here.

You may recall my earlier statements about how we've been conditioned as women: to be the caregivers, the followers, the ones who put others before ourselves. Assertive girls are labeled "bossy." Assertive women? "Bitchy." Thankfully, this is starting to shift, but not quickly enough. Because we're taught to give everything to others, two problems tend to occur:

1. We don't say "no" when we really need to, leading us down a long path of over-accommodation until we finally reach our breaking point.
2. We allow others to "scope creep" on us—slowly taking advantage of our kindness or our discomfort with confrontation.

Before we go any further, let me be absolutely clear: I'm talking about setting boundaries in business, friendships, family dynamics, and everyday negotiations (like trying to get a fair price on your dog's dental cleaning). I am not referring to situations of abuse or assault, where no means no, period. We do not blame victims here, my friend.

Now that that's clear...

Boundaries Are Leadership

You have the beautiful opportunity as a woman to be a leader, not just in your career, but in your life. And women are craving leadership from *other women*. It's different. It's kinder. It's softer. And there's an inherent understanding of what we're all up against when we lead and support each other.

Abby Wambach is one of my favorite celebrities. She was a badass soccer player, breaking records of even men's soccer stars, and she's a humble leader. She talks about *leading from the bench* and her stories from *Wolfpack* resonate with me so much that I often think about leadership in terms of soccer game analogies. Which is weird since I'm about as athletic as a chicken.

Soccer has clear boundaries—goal lines, side lines, penalty areas, time limits—yet within those boundaries, there's immense freedom. Players make creative plays, take risks, and pivot when needed. That's how boundaries work in life, too. When we set clear guardrails for what we will and won't allow, we create space for more ease, creativity, and *actual* freedom. This is what leadership should look like: boundaries for yourself first and then for the people you interact with, so that everyone knows what's acceptable and what's not.

What Are Boundaries, Really?

Nedra Glover Tawwab gives us a great outline of what boundaries are and what they are not. In her book, *Set Boundaries, Find Peace: A Guide to Reclaiming Yourself*, she defines boundaries as *cues to other people on how to treat you*. They help you feel safe, respected, and calm. She identifies them as:

- Safeguards against overextending yourself
- A form of self-care
- Parameters for relationships

- A way to ask others to show up for you
- Clarity
- Safety[1]

And here's a crucial point: boundaries are for you. They're not tools to control others. You can't change someone else's behavior—but you *can* change who you spend time with and what kind of treatment you're willing to accept.

Where Do You Stand with Your Boundaries?

So, how are your boundaries? Do you find that you hold them pretty sacred, or could they use some work? Below, you'll see a few prompts that will help you answer these questions. And as you do, maintain compassion for yourself. You aren't a bad person or wrong in any way. We're always growing, learning, and progressing.

1. On a scale of 1 to 10, how much of yourself do you *want* to share with:
   a. Your partner?
   b. Your family?
   c. Your work peers?
   d. Your friends?
2. Do your boundaries shift depending on who you're interacting with?
3. Do you feel your boundaries are respected?

---

1. Tawwab, N. G. (2021). In *Set boundaries, find peace: A guide to reclaiming yourself.* essay, TarcherPerigee, an imprint of Penguin Random House LLC.

4. Is there someone in your life who continually disrespects your boundaries?
5. If so, how can you reinforce them?
6. How separate do you want your work and personal life to be?
7. What specific boundaries do you need to strengthen?

What If Someone Violates Your Boundary?

So, you've set a boundary...and someone ignores it. What now?

First, remember that clear is kind (thank you, Brené Brown). When addressing a boundary issue, use "I" statements to keep the conversation constructive rather than confrontational. You don't want to trigger defensiveness—you just want to get your needs across.

Here's a simple framework:

1. **State the situation.** *"I noticed that _____. It causes me stress because I feel _____."*
2. **Take responsibility for any part you played.** *(If relevant.)* *"I realize that I may have done _____ in the past."*
3. **Clearly state the boundary.** *"I would appreciate it if we could _____."*
4. **Invite the other person into the solution.** *"How can we make this work for both of us?"*

Keeping your tone calm and casual—while still firm—will help reset the boundary in a way that (hopefully) avoids unnecessary drama.

Burnout often happens because we say yes when we *want* to say no. We take on emotional labor we *don't* have the capacity for. We overextend ourselves out of guilt, obligation, or fear of disappointing others.

Boundaries are how we take back control. They give us permission to prioritize our well-being. They help us protect our energy and create relationships based on mutual respect. If burnout is a cycle, boundaries are the breaks. They stop us from running ourselves into the ground and remind us that *our needs matter, too.*

So, how strong are your boundaries? And where do you need to reinforce them?

19

Breaking Your Personal Burnout Pattern

B reaking the cycle of burnout requires consistent, intentional shifts that support your energy. That means you need a strategy that works with your lifestyle, your personality, and your personal burnout pattern.

Step 1: Identify Your Core Burnout Type

You started this work in Part 2, but if you didn't put it into action yet, now is the time.

Think back on the times when you've felt unreasonably exhausted, disconnected, or like you just couldn't anymore. Then, flip back to Part 2 and review the burnout types. Which ones felt the most familiar? Maybe social burnout drains you the most, but it quickly spirals into emotional exhaustion. Or maybe mental burnout is your default, which eventually leads to physical depletion.

Just as important as recognizing what *is* part of your burnout pattern is identifying what *isn't*. Are there burnout types that don't resonate with you? Maybe you're an introvert who has no trouble saying no to social events, or you're highly attuned to your body, so physical burnout rarely sneaks up on you. The clearer you are about your personal burnout cycle, the more effectively you can break it.

Reflection Questions:

- What burnout type seems to show up first for you?
- Which one tends to spiral into other forms of burnout?
- What emotions do you notice the most when you're burning out?
- What type *isn't* an issue for you?

Once you've identified your core burnout type and how it triggers your personal patterning, it's time to create a personalized approach to breaking the cycle.

Step 2: Choose the Right Strategies for Your Pattern

Each burnout type has different solutions, but not every strategy will resonate with you. Instead of overwhelming yourself with everything at once (hello, fast track to more burnout!), pick one or two small shifts that feel the most doable right now.

To help, here are strategy categories based on burnout type—so you can mix and match based on your burnout pattern. These are just suggestions, feel free to add your own in the spaces provided.

Social Burnout: If People Feel Like Too Much

Pick one or two of ways to support yourself:

- **Create a social Energetic Container.** Designate set times for social activities so you have time to prepare beforehand and recover afterward. Example: A standing Saturday night dinner with friends, knowing you have Sunday to recharge. (More about Energetic Containers in the next chapter!)
- **Audit your relationships.** Are you in *reciprocal* relationships, or do people only reach out when they need something? If a friendship feels draining instead of energizing, it might be time to set firmer boundaries.
- **Schedule alone time like an appointment.** Just as you schedule meetings and events, schedule time for yourself. It's not "free time"—it's *recovery time*.

- **Make social engagements work for you.**
Instead of agreeing to large, high-energy gatherings, suggest lower-stimulation alternatives (e.g., a one-on-one coffee date instead of a loud party).

  - _____
  - _____
  - _____
  - _____

Mental Burnout: If Your Brain Feels Like It's Overloaded

Pick one or two ways to lighten the mental load:

- **Create a reading/listening container.** Set specific times for consuming new information so you don't drown in an endless cycle of input. Example: A "learning hour" in the morning, then switching to output mode (writing, creating, executing).
- **Give your brain playtime.** Do something _unstructured_ that allows your mind to wander— puzzles, coloring, playing music, or even daydreaming. Creativity thrives when you're _not_ forcing it.
- **Take a dopamine detox.** If you constantly refresh your inbox, social media, or news feeds, take intentional breaks from constant stimulation. A 24-hour screen detox or a notification-free weekend can do wonders.

- **Reframe how you view mental work.** If you're *always* consuming information for productivity, you'll burn out. Give yourself permission to read, watch, or learn *for pure enjoyment.*
- **Balance mental effort with movement.** Mental fatigue is real. A 10-minute walk, stretching break, or even just changing rooms can reset your brain.

- _____
- _____
- _____
- _____

Physical Burnout: If Your Body is Running on Empty

Select one or two recovery-focused habits:

- **Honor your rest needs.** Sleep and *true* rest aren't the same. You might be sleeping but not *resting.* Incorporate restorative activities like naps, breathwork, gentle stretching, or time in nature.
- **Schedule recovery activities like appointments.** If bodywork (massage, acupuncture, chiropractic care) helps you, don't wait until you're in pain to book it. Add it to your calendar *before* you hit the wall.
- **Listen to your body's signals.** If you feel exhausted *before* a workout, swap it for stretching

or a walk. Not every workout needs to be high
intensity to be beneficial.

- **Check in with your health.** If fatigue is
persistent, rule out medical causes like vitamin
deficiencies, hormone imbalances, or thyroid issues.
A doctor's visit could be the missing piece.

- _____

- _____

- _____

- _____

Emotional Burnout: If You're Carrying Too Much Emotionally

Choose one or two ways to offload emotional strain:

- **Create an emotional recovery container.**
Set aside time after emotionally demanding tasks
(e.g., client calls, family caregiving, therapy) to
reset. Example: 30 minutes of quiet time after a
stressful workday before engaging with others.
- **Express, don't suppress.** Journaling, voice
notes, or even venting to a trusted friend can help
you process emotions instead of bottling them up.
- **Get creative with your emotions.** Art,
music, movement, or even gardening can help you
release emotional tension in a way that words
sometimes can't.
- **Ground yourself physically.** Emotional
burnout often pulls you _out_ of your body.
Reconnect by walking barefoot in the grass, taking

a hot bath, or using breathing exercises to regulate your nervous system.

- _____
- _____
- _____
- _____

Energetic Burnout: If You Feel Drained from Taking on Too Much

Pick one or two ways to manage your energy flow:

- **Create a reintegration buffer.** After transformational events (like retreats, conferences, or deep conversations), take time alone to process before jumping back into daily life.
- **Protect your energy.** If you're highly sensitive to others' emotions, practice _energetic hygiene._ Visualization techniques (like imagining a protective bubble around you) can help you maintain boundaries.
- **Work with an energy healer.** Reiki, sound healing, medical massage, or even acupuncture can help you release stored energy that's weighing you down.

- **Spend time in nature.** If people and environments feel overwhelming, go somewhere *without* external stimulation—like the beach, a forest, or a quiet park.

- _____
- _____
- _____
- _____

Empathic Burnout: If Caring for Others is Depleting You

Choose one or two ways to set emotional boundaries:

- **Create self-care containers.** Just as you hold space for others, create dedicated time for yourself. Example: If you work in a helping profession, block out non-negotiable *off-hours* to recharge.
- **Find a therapist or support system.** Even the most empathetic people need someone to hold space *for them*. A therapist, coach, or even a trusted friend can help you offload emotional weight.
- **Limit exposure to emotionally draining content.** Doomscrolling the news or taking on others' struggles 24/7 will burn you out. Set limits on how much you consume.

- **Practice detachment, not disconnection.**
Being empathetic doesn't mean absorbing
everyone's pain. Learn to witness without
internalizing. A mantra like *"Their experience is
theirs, not mine"* can help.

- _____
- _____
- _____
- _____

Step 3: Prevent Burnout Before It Starts

Here's where most people get stuck: They try to do too much
at once. But burnout recovery isn't about fixing everything
overnight. It's about making small, sustainable shifts that add
up over time.

The 3-Part Breaking Up With Burnout Commitment

1. **Start small.** Don't try to overhaul your life
overnight. Pick one or two strategies to implement
this week.
2. **Make it part of your routine.** The key to
lasting change is consistency. Set a reminder, block
out time on your calendar, or pair your new habit
with an existing one.
3. **Reassess as needed.** Burnout recovery isn't
linear. If something stops working for you, adjust.
Your needs will shift, and that's okay.

Whether you're actively in burnout or you've been there and you never want to go back, dismantling these patterns is a process, not a quick fix. This isn't about doing more—it's about doing what actually works for you.

You're not meant to run on empty. By aligning your recovery strategies with your specific burnout patterns, you can break the cycle and start living with more energy, ease, and joy.

20

Mastering Your Time and Energy

One of the biggest ways burnout sneaks up on us? How we spend our time and energy. You might think you have no control over your schedule—that your obligations dictate every hour of your day. But the truth is, you have more agency than you think. Even small shifts in how you structure your time and protect your energy can make a huge difference.

And no, I'm not just talking about time management. You can color-code your calendar and optimize your productivity all you want, but if your energy is depleted, no amount of scheduling hacks will save you. The real key is aligning your schedule with your natural energy flow so that your daily and weekly commitments support your well-being rather than drain it.

Even if you work for someone else, you still decide what happens outside of your work hours. That includes setting boundaries—like *not* answering emails at night or declining invitations that don't align with your priorities. But before we start restructuring your time, we need to take an honest look at where it's going right now.

Where Is Your Time Actually Going?

Imagine that, for one week, you had zero responsibilities to anyone but yourself. No obligations. No expectations. How would you choose to spend your time? Write those things down. These are your true priorities—the things that nourish you and align with your values.

Now, take out your calendar. Look at a typical week—last week is ideal, but anything from the past month works too. Be honest: *What did you actually spend your time doing?* Write it down. Go back to your values. You might say that your health is a top priority, but does your schedule reflect that? If not, don't stress, we're going to fix it. For now, just notice it.

To get an even clearer picture, I want you to track your time for the next seven days. This might sound tedious, but trust me, it's eye-opening. Use an app like Toggl or Clockify, or simply keep a notebook at your desk and jot down what you're doing every hour.

As you track your time, pay attention to how you feel while doing each activity. Are you energized or drained? Are you doing something you love, or something you feel obligated to do? Sometimes, we get so caught up in checking things off a list that we don't recognize which activities actually bring us joy.

For example, let's say you spend two hours at your kiddo's soccer practice each week. On paper, that might feel like a chore. But what if, during that time, you're also catching up with another parent you love talking to? What if you use that time to read a book or listen to a podcast you enjoy? Not everything on your schedule is just another task—some of it *feeds* you, and it's important to recognize those moments.

After tracking your time for a week, compare it with your list of true priorities. Where's the mismatch? Are you saying health is important but never making time for movement? Are you craving creativity but spending all your free time doom-scrolling social media?

Before we make adjustments, though, there's one more thing to consider: your energy. Time management alone won't solve burnout. You also need to understand when you work best and how your energy naturally fluctuates throughout the day. That's where an Energetic Inventory comes in.

Understand Your Energy Rhythms

Time management is helpful, but time alone isn't the problem, energy is. You could have a perfectly organized calendar, but if you're trying to power through tasks when your energy is at its lowest, you'll still end up burnt out. That's why understanding your natural rhythms is just as important as managing your time.

The Energetic Inventory helps you work with your body instead of fighting against it. This means identifying when you feel most energized, when you tend to hit a slump, and how you can align your schedule to optimize your natural flow.

Are You an Early Bird or a Night Owl?

I don't know about you, but I'm an early bird. I love sleeping in on weekends, but when it comes to workdays, I'm up and at 'em, ready to put my best work out before noon. By early afternoon, my energy starts to wane—I'm not at my creative best, and my productivity dips. Later in the afternoon, I get a second wind, and I can focus again for a few more hours.

My partner, on the other hand, is a major night owl. If given the chance, he'll stay in bed until nine or ten in the morning. He even has a rule that his team can't call him before 9 a.m. but they also know that he'll be up working until two or three in the morning, powering through projects when most people are winding down or already in bed. That's when he does his best work, hands down.

While not everyone has the flexibility to set their own work hours, understanding when you naturally function best is key to preventing burnout.

Take a moment to reflect on your natural rhythms. *When do you feel most energized? When do you struggle to focus or stay motivated?*

Even if you work a structured 9–5, follow a shift-work schedule, or have kids you shuttle around to activity after activity, you still have some flexibility. You may not be able to shift everything all at once, but a little tweak here and there can make a huge difference in the long run. For now, just start by identifying your patterns.

Track Your Daily Energy Patterns

For the next week, as you track your time, also track your energy levels. You don't need anything fancy—just make a quick note of how you're feeling at different points in the day.

For example, you might jot down something like this:

8:00 AM: Feeling sharp and focused
11:30 AM: Starting to lose steam, need a break
2:00 PM: Brain fog, struggling to concentrate
4:30 PM: Second wind, feeling productive again
9:00 PM: Exhausted, ready for bed

After a few days, patterns will start to emerge. You'll notice when your energy peaks and when it dips—and that's powerful information, especially when you layer it in with the activities you're doing at those times. Since your energy can be impacted by the time of day *and* by the activity you're doing or the people you're around, you'll need to exercise some discernment. Just remember, this is all about exploring and experimenting. Get curious and notice what comes up.

Factor In Weekly & Monthly Energy Cycles

Daily energy isn't the only thing that matters—our energy also fluctuates throughout the week and month.

Mondays may feel sluggish as you shift from weekend mode into work mode. Or maybe you're one of those "hit the ground running" people and Mondays are your best days. Some of us hit our stride mid-week and schedule our meetings and client work during that period. Friday could be best for wrapping up loose ends instead of starting new projects.

If you menstruate, your monthly cycle also affects your energy levels. You'll want to track your own patterns, of course, but this is what the science says about the female hormonal cycle:

- **Follicular phase (after your period)** – High energy, great for brainstorming and starting new things.
- **Ovulation phase** – Peak energy, best for collaboration, social events, and speaking up.
- **Luteal phase (before your period)** – Lower energy, ideal for admin work and tying up loose ends.
- **Menstrual phase** – Rest and reflection; give yourself more grace and alone time if possible.

Awareness of these patterns and how they play out in your own life allows you to adjust your schedule proactively—instead of constantly feeling like you're running on empty. Once you identify your natural energy flow on a daily, weekly and monthly basis, you can start aligning how you spend your time accordingly.

Energetic Containers

Traditional time blocking never worked for me. It felt too rigid, too much pressure to fit into perfectly scheduled blocks with no room for flow. So, instead, I created Energetic Containers—a flexible way to structure your time based on your natural energy rhythms.

Energetic Containers are designated time periods where you group similar tasks together based on your energy levels. Instead of assigning rigid time slots, these containers allow flexibility within structure, so you can move tasks around without completely derailing your day. If mornings are your prime time, schedule deep work (like writing, problem-solving, or strategic planning) in the early hours when your brain is firing on all cylinders. If you hit a slump in the afternoon, use that time for lower-energy work, like answering emails, organizing your workspace, or taking a movement break to reset. If you get a second wind in the evening, save that time for creative work or personal projects rather than forcing yourself into bed early.

While it's not always possible to plan your schedule exactly the way you'd like, using Energetic Containers helps prevent burnout by reducing task switching, decision fatigue, and misaligned energy use. And on those days when you have a big deadline or a mandatory work event is scheduled smack in the middle of your menstrual phase, well, you'll be that much more resilient because you're not constantly hovering on the brink of burnout.

How to Create Your Energetic Containers

1. **Start with a Clean Slate** – Imagine your schedule is completely clear. What are the activities you love doing? This could include workouts, journaling, client calls, creative work, brunch with your besties, playtime with your kiddo...whatever brings you joy and fills your cup.

2. **Factor in Logistics** – Consider external factors like time zones, team schedules, meetings, standing commitments, and the patterns you noticed from your energy inventory. These are things that shape your day or week.

3. **Group Similar Activities** – Look for patterns in your tasks and organize them into containers based on shared importance or energy requirements.

These containers aren't hard and fast, and you can move them around each week. Personally, I love to fiddle with my calendar for the following week on Friday mornings to block out time or shift containers around depending on what feels right.

Here are some examples of Energetic Containers I work with each week:

- **Writing container** – This could include book writing, working on blogs, social media content, or newsletters.

- **Networking container** – Engaging on social media, reaching out in the DM's to send personalized messages to connections, meeting for coffee chats with my network partners, or inviting folks to an upcoming event via personalized emails.
- **Organization container** – Getting my calendar in shape, making personal and medical appointments, business admin.
- **Family container** – Dinner time, family connection, movies, and weekend fun.
- **Call container** – Sales calls, client calls, meetings.
- **Movement container** – Working out, walking the dog, bodywork.

These containers aren't rigid, you can move them around weekly to reflect changes in workload, energy, and personal priorities. And if you menstruate, consider adjusting your containers based on your cycle, as your energy levels will naturally fluctuate.

If possible, schedule your meetings in containers on the day(s) of the week when you know you're at your best. Some people love a Monday morning meeting. Others love to catch up at the end of the day. Figure out what works best for you, and make an effort to shift things as needed.

As you think about these Energetic Containers, please make sure you are aligning how you are spending your time with what matters most to you. The whole point of this work is to unplug from the shoulds and expectations that fuel burnout.

I'm not helping you clean up your calendar so you can fill it with more that drains you!

Days of the Week Energies

Now, because I can't help myself, I've got to weave a little magic into this. If you want to take energy alignment a step further, consider structuring your tasks around the natural energies of the days of the week. Each day carries a unique rhythm, and aligning your work with these energies can create more ease and flow in your schedule.

Monday

Monday is full of Divine Feminine energy and is ruled by the Moon. This is the perfect day to develop ideas, tap into your intuition, and get really creative. If your clients/customers are women, Mondays are a great day to share stories with them on your blog or on social media.

Tuesday

Tuesday carries fiery, ambitious energy, ruled by Mars, the planet of action. Quite simply, this is your get-shit-done day. Use Tuesdays to make bold decisions, tackle big projects, and have difficult conversations you've been putting off. It's also a powerful day for exercising leadership and standing in your authority.

Wednesday

Wednesdays are ruled by Mercury, the planet of communication, making this the best day for sales calls, networking, writing, and knowledge-sharing. Whether you're drafting a newsletter, pitching an idea, or learning something new, Wednesday's energy supports clear, effective communication and expansion of your skill set.

Thursday

Thursday is ruled by Jupiter, the planet of growth, success, and abundance. This day is ideal for career moves, financial planning, and business development. Use Thursdays for strategy, visioning, balancing your books, planning your next steps, and brainstorming bold new ideas.

Friday

Fridays are all about love, pleasure, and relationships, ruled by Venus. This is the perfect day to connect with others—whether that's through networking, social time, or deepening relationships with loved ones. It's also an ideal day for self-care and honoring yourself before heading into the weekend.

Saturday

Saturdays, ruled by Saturn, are excellent for personal growth, self-discipline, and transformation. This is the perfect day for deep reflection, setting personal goals, or engaging in activities that challenge you—like a workout, a creative project, or a class that stretches your skills.

Sunday

Sunday, ruled by the Sun, carries strong Divine Masculine energy—full of potential, motivation, and renewal. This is an excellent day for vision work, planning for the week ahead, tidying up your calendar, and engaging in creative projects that inspire you.

As you're thinking about your ideal schedule, make sure that it includes some sort of "weekend." We all need a break. I choose to take Saturdays and Sundays off, and I encourage you to take two back-to-back days off a week. Perhaps this means you take Sundays and Mondays off because you meet with clients or show houses on Saturdays. Make your days off work for you and be sure to take them. It's just another way to combat burnout by making space for play, relaxation, and the things that bring you joy.

Protecting Your Schedule

Creating an ideal schedule is one thing—protecting it is another. Without firm boundaries, even the best-planned containers can get hijacked by other people's priorities, unexpected demands, and, let's be honest, our own habits of over-committing. Setting boundaries with your time isn't about being rigid or unkind; it's about respecting your energy and capacity so that you don't fall back into burnout.

One of the biggest struggles people face when protecting their time is saying no. If you struggle with this, remember that every yes is a no to something else. When you agree to one more work commitment, you might be saying no to rest, exercise, or time with your family. Boundaries with your time are not selfish—they are a necessary part of maintaining your energy. If you find yourself hesitating to turn something down, try shifting your language. Instead of saying, "I don't have time," reframe it as, "That doesn't fit into my schedule right now." Instead of squeezing something in just to accommodate someone else, try, "I'd love to, but I don't have the bandwidth for it." These subtle changes help reinforce that your time is valuable, and it's okay to prioritize yourself.

Another way to protect your schedule is to block off time for breaks and recharge moments—because if you don't, those moments will get filled with distractions or last-minute obligations. Treat rest like an essential appointment. That means setting aside time for an actual lunch break instead of inhaling a sandwich while checking emails, scheduling small afternoon resets like a quick walk or stretch session, and carving out evening wind-down time free from work notifications. If a break is on your calendar, respect it the same way you would a meeting with your boss. The only difference? *You're the boss of your energy.*

Boundaries also matter when it comes to handling last-minute requests and interruptions. If you feel like your day constantly gets derailed by other people's needs, setting clear communication boundaries can help. For work, that might mean establishing response times, such as only checking emails at specific hours rather than being available around the clock. In your social life, it could mean letting people know you need a heads-up before making plans so you're not caught off guard. Even in family and close relationships, you can set boundaries by being upfront about when you need space instead of feeling obligated to respond to every call or message immediately. The key is remembering that you don't need to be available 24/7. People will adjust to your boundaries—as long as you uphold them.

Another essential layer of protecting your schedule is setting digital boundaries. Our phones are designed to demand our attention constantly, and if you're always reacting to notifications, you're letting external forces dictate your day. Turning off non-essential notifications can be a game changer, especially for work apps like Slack or email that don't always require immediate responses. Setting your phone to "Do Not Disturb" during focused work periods helps reinforce the habit of being present with your tasks rather than reacting to every buzz and ping. You can also establish personal "office hours" for checking messages—deciding when (and if) you'll respond, rather than feeling obligated to be reachable at all times. The more intentional you are about where your attention goes, the easier it will be to keep burnout at bay.

21

Rest, You Dehydrated Goddess!

Phew! We've made it this far, and now it's time for some deep, soulful rest—the kind that doesn't just recharge your body, but restores you at the core. Because rest and sleep? Not the same thing.

You've probably had nights where you technically *slept*, but still woke up feeling like a zombie. Those nights when you toss and turn or you struggle with nightmares and anxiety-fueled images running through your head. Or maybe you *did* get enough sleep, but instead of feeling refreshed, you launched into the day like you were already behind. That's not true rest. Also, when's the last time you drank some water? Go take a sip. I'll wait.

We live in a productivity-obsessed culture where rest is treated as a luxury instead of a necessity. Toxic capitalism tells us we have to be constantly grinding, constantly available, constantly *doing*. But as you know, by now burnout thrives in a world where rest is treated as optional.

I'm fascinated by Sandra Dalton-Smith, M.D.'s seven types of rest. I think they pair perfectly with my six types of burnout. According to Dr. Dalton-Smith, we don't just need more rest; we need the right kind of rest:

- **Physical rest**—Whether active (like yoga or stretching) or passive (like naps or massage), your body needs downtime.
- **Mental rest**—Taking short breaks throughout the day and slowing your thoughts instead of running on overdrive.
- **Sensory rest**—Stepping away from screens, bright lights, and constant stimulation.
- **Creative rest**—Reconnecting with nature, music, art, and anything that *fills* you instead of *drains* you.
- **Emotional rest**—Expressing your emotions openly, without filtering yourself to make others comfortable.
- **Social rest**—Spending time with people who uplift and restore you, instead of those who drain you.
- **Spiritual rest**—Connecting with something bigger than yourself, whether that's through faith, meditation, or community.[1]

It's easy to invest time in one or two forms of rest and neglect

---

1. Saundra Dalton-Smith, "The 7 Types of Rest That Every Person Needs," ideas.ted.com (TED, January 6, 2021), https://ideas.ted.com/the-7-types-of-rest-that-every-person-needs/.

the others. Maybe you prioritize sleep, but never give yourself creative rest. Maybe you get physical rest but neglect emotional rest because you're too busy tending to others. Yet, sometimes, the rest we need is the one we're "too busy" to take. Consider which type of rest you actually need, not just the one that fits neatly into your schedule.

Rest is the antidote to burnout. And it's not a sign of weakness. In fact, resting is a great way to give the middle finger to the patriarchy. So take the break. Claim your space. Give yourself permission to rest without guilt.

Because, my friend, resting is resistance—and you deserve it.

Conclusion

I promised myself I wouldn't be in that place again—running on fumes, scatter-brained, existing on coffee and insomnia. And yet, there I was, driving around in a haze of last-minute holiday errands, thinking exactly that: *I promised myself I wouldn't be here again.*

I was writing a book about burnout, damn it. I knew all the tricks, had all the strategies. I knew better. And yet...here I was. My partner had left one company, expecting to start a new position, only for the opportunity to fall through. Financially, we were fine, but the mental and emotional strain of his four months without work weighed on us both. My son had recently started hormone replacement therapy, making his transition all that more real and demanding a deeper commitment from me in supporting my boy through this change. Christmas was days away, and I was looking at the reality of having to put down my beloved dog, Pluto. (We did, in fact, have to say goodbye.)

I was taking care of everything and everyone—except myself. The weight of it all pulled me back into burnout.

So why am I telling you this? Because, my friend, I never want you to feel like you've failed if you've broken up with burnout and it creeps back in. It doesn't mean you're back at square one. It means you're human.

Here's the truth about doing this work:

1. The level of burnout you experience is never as deep again because you know how to manage it,
2. It takes a lot more to burn you out than before, and
3. When it does happen, you have a clearer path to getting out of it.

For me, it took a job loss, a transitioning child, the impending loss of a pet, holiday chaos, and end-of-year exhaustion to tip me back into burnout. That's a lot. And maybe, at some point, you'll find yourself here again, too.

That's okay.

The goal isn't to eliminate burnout from your life forever. The goal is to recognize it sooner, navigate it faster, and recover with more ease and self-compassion.

So, keep going. Keep making the changes that support you. Keep showing up for yourself.

We *can* do this. We *can* revolutionize our lives. And one by one, as we reclaim our energy and our well-being, we'll inspire others to do the same. And maybe, just maybe, burnout will one day be a thing of the past.

Until then, take care of yourself.

Resources for Further Support

Need More Support?

Burnout recovery doesn't end when you close the back cover of this book. If you'd like more tools, community, and support, visit MeganWinkler.com.

There, you'll find free resources, deeper readings, and ways to stay connected to this work—and most importantly, to yourself.

Tools and Techniques

The Pomodoro® Method

A simple, structured approach to improving focus and productivity.

Learn more at:
francescocirillo.com/products/the-pomodoro-technique

Internal Family Systems (IFS)

A transformative, evidence-based approach to inner healing and self-connection.

Learn more at: ifs-institute.com

Guided Meditations Playlist

Curated meditation practices to support nervous system regulation, emotional recovery, and mental clarity.

Explore the playlist on YouTube: Meditation Playlist

Support for Safety

Domestic Violence Hotline

If you or someone you know needs help, the National Domestic Violence Hotline is available 24/7.

Call 800-799-7233 or visit thehotline.org.

Acknowledgments

I would like to express my deepest gratitude to my family and friends for their unwavering support and endless encouragement as I poured my heart and soul into these pages, especially my partner in everything, Mike. Seriously, I couldn't do any of the work I do without you. Thank you for shouldering the extra household labor with me, providing me with a sounding board for new ideas, and laughing with me through life! Thank you also to my son, Danny, who teaches me something new every day.

Many thanks to Michelle Fishering, my book coach and head cheerleader, for your guidance and careful reading and rereading (and then rereading again). Thank you for believing in this book as much as I do! Thank you also to Johanna Oosterwijk, my Reiki mentor, for supporting me on my energetic healing journey and passing down knowledge to me with such love, safety, and warmth.

I'd be terribly remiss if I didn't shout-out my ever-supportive and clients. Of course, I have to thank my Ecosystem Energy Fam: Darnell, Erika, Sandy, Robin, Mekayla, and Rachel. Thanks for continuing to light a fire under my butt!

Finally, many thanks to Abby Wambach, who may never read this book but who inspired me to create my own form of leadership and look at the challenges we face as women in a completely different way—*Wolfpack* inspired me so much through this journey!

And of course, thank YOU. Thank you for reading this book, sharing this book, and coming on this journey with me.

About the Author

Megan Winkler is a business consultant, historian, and Reiki Master. She holds a master's degree in military history and an MBA in women in leadership, and loves supporting animal rescue organizations. Megan blends her certifications in Reiki and meditation with her expertise in intuitive guidance and strategic planning to help high-achieving and neurodivergent women create clarity, consistency, and sustainability in their careers and lives.

With a passion for empowering ADHD and highly sensitive people, Megan incorporates astrology, tarot, and her signature Energetic Containers framework into her work, offering a magical yet practical approach to personal and professional growth.

When she's not helping her clients align their lives with their unique strengths and cosmic blueprints, she's spending time with her husband and family in North Texas.